Richard Hittleman's

YOGA
FOR
HEALTH

Based on the
Independent Television Series

Hamlyn
London · New York · Sydney · Toronto

Until very recently, to the vast majority of people in the West, Yoga connoted only a remote mysticism practised by Eastern holy men, involving such uncomfortable activities as lying on beds of nails !

A few people, however, took the trouble to study and analyse Yoga thought and techniques and realised that Hatha—or Physical—Yoga provided a system of exercising the body and quietening the mind which had immediate and practical benefits in the promotion of health, weight control and relaxation from the strains of modern living.

One man in particular has made it his life study to examine the Yoga techniques and to translate them to the needs of present-day living. This man, Richard Hittleman, first learned of Yoga exercises when he was an eight-year-old child on the East Coast of America. Today, with 20 years of teaching behind him he is the foremost Yoga instructor in the United States and it has been estimated that through his work no less than ten million Americans have become familiar with the basic principles of Yoga.

It was an East Indian employee of his parents who first initiated the young Richard into Yoga exercises. He soon found these exercises were both relaxing and revitalising. He was strongly attracted by the serenity and peaceful nature of his teacher and realised that this was a result of the exercises.

During the whole of his educational period he became engrossed in research on the subject of Yoga and after obtaining his Master's Degree from Columbia University Teachers' College, he carried out post-graduate work at the American Academy of Asian Studies in San Francisco.

Since then he has travelled considerably and studied techniques at first hand in the East. As a result of this he has developed a unique system of Yoga instruction which is now to be seen in his television series YOGA FOR HEALTH. Despite the remarkable growth of his work in the United States, Richard Hittleman's teachings have hitherto been confined to that country. Now, through the medium of television, they are being made available in other countries, where the problems of modern living are just as severe and where the need for an effective and permanent remedy is as acute.

YOGA FOR HEALTH has been filmed and produced in LONDON and the exercises have been carefully chosen to combat the strains inherent in twentieth century society.

HOWARD KENT and HAROLD ORTON
Producers, "Yoga for Health"

PRINCIPLES OF RICHARD HITTLEMAN'S YOGA INSTRUCTION

For many thousands of people, dreams of a new life, a return to second youth, a beautiful, strong and trim body which radiates health and vitality, and wonderful peace of mind, have come true through my Yoga instruction. There is no reason why any or all of these things should not be yours. You have these things within you *now*, although you may be unaware or have forgotten this fact. I will show you how to awaken these wonderful hidden forces which lie asleep within you and make them work for you *24 hours a day*.

If you have been following my TV programmes for some time, you already know the great and profound truth of the preceding paragraph. If you are a new student, you will very quickly learn that you have embarked on a most fascinating adventure which can lead you to the pinnacle of physical and metal well-being!

THE WISDOM OF THE YOGA SAGES

Yoga is the 'grandfather' of all of the systems and methods of 'self-improvement'. It has been used for many centuries by people throughout the world to gain new life for their bodies and minds. You can only appreciate how great was the wisdom of the brilliant men who devised these marvellous physical and mental exercises when you actually practise Yoga. In certain ways, they seemed to know much more about how to make our bodies function as the beautiful, precision instruments they are, than we do today. The wisdom of these exercises, combined with the wonderful discoveries of modern science regarding the preservation of our health and youth, will enable you to 'design' the type of body you want. And the beauty of my Yoga method is that you need no gadgets, gimmicks or apparatus to accomplish this! If this sounds almost too good to be true, it is simply because you are not aware of the tremendous power of your body to *recondition* itself when you give it the proper stimulus. And this stimulus will be your Yoga practice and certain dynamic principles regarding nutrition—that is, your eating habits.

WHAT YOGA IS NOT

From time to time I hear someone say, "But Yoga comes from India, therefore it is something 'foreign' and I don't see how we can make use of it." Of course this is foolishness. It is like saying, "I don't want to listen to the music of Bach because he was a German," or it is like someone in India declaring "We don't want to use electricity, because Thomas Edison was an American." Yoga is universal. It is a priceless gift from the East and its benefits are available to all of us who would accept them.

It is very tragic that many of us, not knowing the facts, have for many years confused Yogis (a person who practises 'Yoga' is a 'Yogi') with a certain class of people in India who are known as Fakirs. Fakirs have gained extraordinary control of their senses, but use this control to subject their bodies to abnormal conditions. For example, they sit on the famous 'bed of nails', stick pins and swords into their bodies, allow themselves to be 'buried alive' and perform other such 'supernatural' feats. They are generally persons of low mentality, and they perform these supernatural things for money, food, favours and so forth. These Fakirs should never be confused with Yogis. Nor do snake charmers or Indian Rope trick practitioners have anything to do with Yoga. Yoga is a method of *natural* development for body and mind and a true Yogi will never permit anything harmful or unnatural to be done to his body or mind.

Finally, there is the question of 'religion'. I am often asked, "Is Yoga a religion?" My answer is, "Definitely not!". For us, Yoga is a dynamic system of physical exercise and a practical and valuable philosophy to apply to everyday life; in short, Yoga is a *way of life* and everyone, regardless of his religion, can benefit greatly from any one or all aspects of Yoga.

THE POWER ASLEEP WITHIN YOU

Now let's talk about the important principles which will enable *you* to get the very most out of your Yoga practice *each day*, whether you're doing it by yourself, or practising with me.

You undoubtedly were (or soon will be) most delighted with the progress you made in your first 15 days of Yoga practice. *Your body itself wants the very things you would like it to have!* Trimness, strength, beauty, poise, balance, flexibility, vitality, radiance, serenity and optimism are all within your grasp. Your body has within it, at all times, the wonderful power to recondition itself and bring them out. But this power (which in Yoga we refer to as the 'Life-Force') has to be stimulated and activated so that it can accomplish this "bringing out". I am not going to go too deeply into the explanation of how or why this miraculous Life-Force works. We will leave this for our later discussions. The point is, that it *does* work the moment you begin to stimulate it through your Yoga exercises and understand about "life" foods. It seems to be universally true that people who undertake to perform the Yoga exercises and pay attention to their diets as I instruct them, stimulate the 'Life-Force' almost immediately. The body begins to recondition itself, producing all of the wonderful results which I know you want. *Stop looking for gadgets and gimmicks! Real health and beauty comes from within. Therefore, START YOUR YOGA EXERCISES AND PAY ATTENTION TO NUTRITION NOW. The new life you seek is nearer than you dream!*

FROM 4 TO 80

I have been very encouraged by the wide age range of people who join us in our TV programmes. It is no exaggeration to say that children from 4 years old to senior citizens beyond 80 practise with us daily. Children love to manipulate their bodies; it seems that the exercises present a challenge to them. I know that the Yoga movements help children to grow properly and make their bodies firm and strong. Parents should encourage their children to learn and practise these movements, for once they are learned they become a lifetime habit. Don't you wish you had been taught these marvellous exercises when you were very young? As children grow older, Yoga practice will aid them in school; the postures calm them when necessary, and also seem to produce an alertness and clarity of mind that is most important in their studies. So make sure that they do the exercises with you. At the other extreme, I find that senior citizens, well along in years but young in spirit, very quickly begin to regain many of the characteristics of youth as they practise Yoga. This is because the 'Life-Force' is always within us and can be activated at any age and under almost any conditions. Therefore, elderly persons who are stiff, tight, cramped and tense, begin to loosen up and, as this happens, they naturally begin to feel 'younger'; they become more active and are able to enjoy life to a much greater degree.

It is of absolutely no importance how 'stiff' or 'out of condition' you think you are or how 'well' you are able to do these exercises in the first few months of your practice. Do not be discouraged if you do not have the flexible body of an athlete, or think that you cannot benefit from Yoga because of your 'stiffness'. You will be making a great mistake. And our senior citizens prove the truth of this when, regardless of their age or physical condition, they begin these mild, gentle stretches which require so little energy and effort. Very quickly, they learn that each day they are able to go a little further, loosen themselves a little more, gain a little better control. Soon they are amazed at the results. In other words, Yoga is *progressive. Once you begin practising, you can only get better!* With some, this progress is quicker than with others, but the rapidity of progress should be of no concern to us. Our progress may be a little slower than another's, but it is the law of nature that there is always steady improvement. Each day you will become more aware of the marvellous power of the 'Life-Force' and how it is reconditioning and building a new body for you.

Between these extreme ages, that is, children and senior citizens, we have people of all ages and from every walk of life who practise Yoga for many reasons. These include girls and women who want to trim and firm their bodies; rid themselves of flabbiness and excess weight; gain poise, beauty, and radiance; men who wish to gain strength and vitality and relieve themselves of nervous tension and fatigue. The reasons for which Yoga is practised and the effects of the exercises are far too many to be listed here. They would require an entire book. But you will soon know for yourself what can be accomplished when the 'Life-Force' is activated.

YOGA AND YOUR DOCTOR

Yoga exercises *are never to be used as a substitute for medical treatment.* If you are ill or have a history of a serious illness and you are in doubt as to how these exercises will affect you, then you must see your doctor. He is the only person who is qualified to tell you the type of exercises you may undertake. However, it has been my experience that doctors are almost always in favour of having their patients remain active, and the mildness of Yoga makes it particularly advantageous for those who must not exercise strenuously. I have had many doctors in my classes. Their reaction is extremely favourable toward Yoga as a form of exercise. If you doctor is not familiar with Yoga, show him the exercises in this book. From the doctor's standpoint, the great value of Yoga lies in the number of areas of the body which are stretched and strengthened with a minimum expenditure of energy.

THE IMPORTANCE OF SLOW MOTION

I have often said during my TV programmes that "20 minutes of Yoga is worth an hour of ordinary exercise." And along with this, I have told you that "one movement in Yoga is better than 10 movements in the usual 'setting-up' exercises." I believe that you have already been able to determine the truth of this for yourself. The principle behind these statements is the *slow-motion* movement and the frequent *holds* of Yoga exercises. It is this slow-motion moving and the holding which enables the muscles, tendons and ligaments to truly stretch, strengthen, become taut and firm, and the joints to become flexible. As far as we are concerned in Yoga, the usual quick 1-2, 1-2, movements of ordinary exercise have very little value, since we are not interested in quickening the pulse and heart, and perspiring. Why place a strain on your heart and throw away your energy when it would seem that the benefits of exercise should consist of *relieving tension* and *strain*, and conserving *energy*? And there is another extremely important reason for this *slow-motion and holding* principle of Yoga. We find that this type of movement tends frequently to stimulate and aid in the proper functioning of the *internal organs and glands*. Don't you find this an extremely fascinating concept? It is a factor that no ordinary exercise considers! So keep this slow-motion principle in mind while you're practising your Yoga. You will hear me telling you to move slowly over and over again during my TV programmes, because I know how valuable it is for you to learn to move slowly and gain real control over your body in these days when life moves at a killing tempo. During our practice we have plenty of time to move slowly since it is seldom necessary to perform any exercise more than 3 to 5 times.

YOU'RE MORE BEAUTIFUL THAN YOU THINK

"*Think gracefully!*" It is true that "the body is the temple of the spirit". It is also true that you *are* beautiful since you were 'made' in the image of everything that is beauty and truth. If you *think* it, *know* it and *act* it, you will *become* it. No matter what your physical condition, nor how stiff, tense, awkward or clumsy you *think* you are, you must exchange these thoughts for those of grace, poise, beauty, harmony and balance. The Wisdom and Life-Force within you will gradually respond to this stimulus and you will find your body gaining these positive attributes. During our Yoga practice on TV, and regardless of what you are doing during the day, move your body as if you were dancing in a ballet. Never laugh at, or reprimand yourself for being clumsy or awkward. When I tell you to 'sit' or 'stand' gracefully and you find it difficult to do so, do your best. If you feel like laughing for making what you think is a 'clumsy' movement, try to control yourself immediately. In re-educating your body you are training a 'spoiled' child. It will get away with whatever it can and it likes to make you laugh at it to show you that *it* is the master and *you* are its servant and that it can do whatever it likes. You must reverse this position. *You* must become the master and make the body respond to *your* wishes. You train a child, especially a 'spoiled' child, by being gentle, but firm and forceful. The same idea must prevail in re-educating your body. Think gracefully, be firm, forceful, and confident, and always feel you are in control.

ASSISTING OTHERS

It is important to note that you can utilize the new force and power that you will gain through your Yoga practice to assist others in living a more healthy life, both physically and mentally. Your relatives and friends are certain to notice that a very positive change is occurring within you and will question you about this change. If you wish to tell them about your Yoga practice, do so with restraint and intelligence. Do not force the idea on them or appear over-anxious for anyone to practise Yoga. When you maintain a calm and restrained manner in explaining Yoga, you will find that people are all the more interested in listening and then practising. Every person to whom you introduce Yoga will be eternally grateful. If another person ever pokes fun or scoffs at you for practising Yoga, you can be sure it is because he secretly envies you. It has been my experience that many so-called 'friends' really are envious of your efforts and will-power in self-improvement because they themselves don't have it. But you can be sure that their ridicule will very quickly cease when they see the unmistakable signs of what is happening to your body. So never allow a weak friend to deter you from your self-improvement practises.

ANOTHER ASPECT OF YOGA

Another vital way to use the power which will be made available to you through the Yoga exercises, is to 'project' this force throughout the entire world with the thought of *Harmony* and *Peace* behind it. This is accomplished simply by sitting down for one minute in the Lotus or Cross-Legged posture, either before or after your Yoga practice period, and sending out postive thoughts while performing the slow, rhythmic breathing of the Complete Breath. This technique will prove to be most effective, and the more power you project, the more force you will find that you yourself are receiving. This entire procedure results eventually in a great internal security and peace of mind. There are very great rewards for your careful and patient practice of Yoga.

Along these lines you may know that there are 'mental' as well as physical exercises in Yoga. Just as these physical techniques are designed to help you gain health, control and development of *your* body, so are the mental techniques of Yoga designed to gain health, control and development of your mind and emotions. We will not go deeply into the mental techniques in this book. However, I want you to be aware that there *are* mental exercises, that they are very practical and natural, that they form a very important part of Yoga and that we *will* be getting to them soon. But first, I want you to see what physical Yoga can do for your body. I want you to gain the strength, beauty, health, confidence and new life that comes from this practice. I want you to notice how every activity in your daily life improves. Be sure to join me as often as possible in our TV practice and use this book as your guide.

AS YOU PROCEED

With each day of Yoga practice, you will find yourself making new advances. It is important at this point of our study that I explain in a little more detail some of the things that you can expect as you go forward with Yoga. You are stretching and strengthening many areas of your body that have probably not been methodically exercised in many years. This may result in some minor discomforts; slight aches and pains can occur from time to time, and it is important for you to understand that this is the natural course of removing tensions and stiffness and of rebuilding your body. If you have days when you experience such minor discomforts, you must simply practise very easily or even temporarily discontinue the particular exercises that are causing the strain. In a day or two, this uncomfortable feeling will pass and then you can continue your practice. If you follow this procedure, and never strain or overdo, you will find that it is possible to impart new strength and life to even the most difficult and stubborn areas of your body.

SPECIAL PROBLEMS

Many students have requested special information to help overcome specific physical problems. In complying with these numerous requests, I have included in this book two pages of important tables which indicate combinations of exercises that can be emphasized for various conditions and parts of the body. However, in practising any one or more groups of these exercises which you may select, do not neglect the remaining postures. For example, if you wish to reduce weight in a particular part of your body, you can consult the tables and emphasize the exercises advised. *But weight control is a matter of the proper functioning of many organs and glands throughout the body.* Therefore, to help insure the correct functioning of such organs and glands, it is necessary to learn *and practise* as many as possible of the exercises contained in the book.

THE NEW LIFE THAT WILL SOON BE YOURS

By using this book as a guide, and practising with me seriously during my TV instruction, you can expect to accomplish the following:

(1) Trim, firm, and strengthen your entire body.

(2) Rid yourself of flabbiness and excess weight.

(3) Gain flexibility and elasticity; relieve stiffness and tightness.

(4) Gain poise, beauty, balance, radiance, grace and self-confidence.

(5) Relieve tension, nervousness and insomnia.

(6) Increase energy and vitality.

(7) Improve in everything you do, physically as well as mentally.

If you would like to write about your progress with the exercises, or about anything relating to Yoga, I will be most happy to hear from you. May I wish you every success in the wonderful new life that will be yours through—

''Y O G A   F O R   H E A L T H''

RICHARD L. HITTLEMAN

SEVEN IMPORTANT RULES FOR YOUR YOGA PRACTICE

(1) Always practise easily and carefully. There is no point in straining to accomplish more or go further, since Yoga is progressive. If you practise regularly, as I advise you, your progress will be steady and sure, and you will never experience any soreness.

(2) Practise with me as often as possible during the TV programmes. Then, if you wish, you may practise once again at any time later on in the day. You may practise any exercises you desire and spend from 20 to 45 minutes doing them. It is seldom necessary to practise more than twice each day to experience maximum benefits for our purposes.

(3) People often like to practise with one or more friends or relatives. This is a good idea, providing that discipline is maintained so that the practice period is not spent in chatting and watching one another. Many people prefer to practise alone. If you can, always find a quiet spot, indoors or outdoors for practice. This is not always possible and you will simply have to find a place or wait for a time when there are the least number of distractions. It is important to have a calm and serene state of mind when practising.

(4) Your practice place should have a good supply of fresh air. Remove all tight or confining clothing, including belt, watch, shoes and eye-glasses. For some exercises you will need your watch or clock, so keep it handy. Use the same mat or towel for your practice each day and do not allow it to be used for any other purpose. Have as little food as possible in your stomach when you practise.

(5) Start paying attention to your NUTRITION *now*. I cannot overemphasize the importance of knowing the value (what is 'alive' and what is 'dead') of what you are eating, as discussed on my TV series.

(6) Keep a separate notebook for your Yoga practice. You will want to write down many things you learn on our programmes, as well as making your own notes of things that come up during your practice.

(7) Your Yoga practice period will be the most important time you devote each day to your physical and mental self-improvement and well-being. Therefore, always be serious and careful as you practise, doing all the movements exactly as I teach them to you, with a great sense of beauty, poise, balance, grace and rhythm. Be confident and *know* that you will accomplish all of the things I have told you are possible through Yoga.

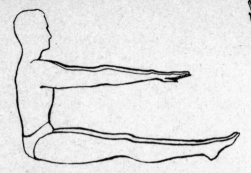

1. SIT WITH LEGS STRAIGHT OUT BE-FORE YOU. _SLOWLY_ AND GRACE-FULLY RAISE ARMS.

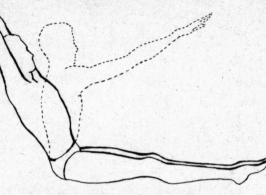

2. _SLOWLY_ BRING ARMS UP AND BACK AND LEAN BACKWARD SEV-ERAL INCHES.

1. LEG PULLS

COUNT 5 FOR ALL MOVEMENTS
— PERFORM 3 TO 5 TIMES

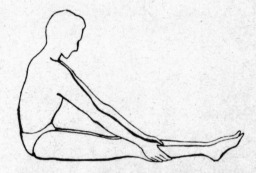

3. _SLOWLY_ COME FORWARD AND TAKE HOLD OF WHATEVER PART OF LEGS YOU CAN REACH WITH-OUT A STRAIN.

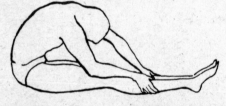

4. GENTLY PULL TRUNK DOWNWARD AS FAR AS YOU CAN WITHOUT STRAIN AND HOLD.

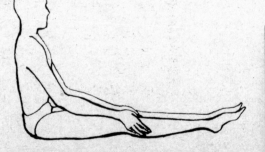

5. RELEASE LEGS AND _SLOWLY_ STRAIGHTEN UP. RELAX—REPEAT.

LEG PULLS

You can expect to:
Reduce flabbiness and remove excess weight by firming the LEGS, THIGHS and BUTTOCKS.
Remove tension and stiffness throughout the LEGS, BACK and NECK. Strengthen and develop the LEGS and BACK.

2. BACKWARD BEND

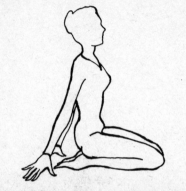

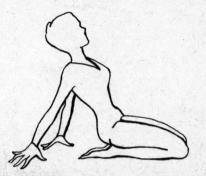

1. SIT ON HEELS. KEEP KNEES ON THE FLOOR AND TOUCH FINGER TIPS OR HANDS TO THE FLOOR ON EITHER SIDE.

2. _SLOWLY_ MOVE HANDS OR FINGER TIPS BACK TO A COMFORTABLE DISTANCE BEHIND YOU.

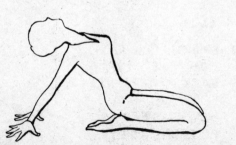

> **BACKWARD BEND**
>
> **You can expect to:**
> Firm and develop the ABDOMEN, CHEST and BUST.
> Remove tension and stiffness and strengthen the TOES, FEET, ANKLES and NECK.

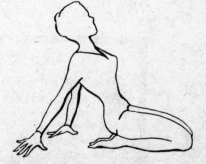

3. _SLOWLY_ RAISE TRUNK TO FORM AN ARCH; DROP HEAD BACK BUT STAY SEATED ON HEELS. HOLD THIS POSITION.

4. _SLOWLY_ RELAX TRUNK. REST IN THE POSITION OF (2). REPEAT.

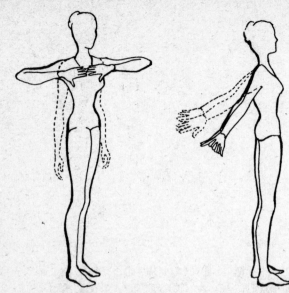

3. CHEST EXPANSION

1. STAND EASILY AND ERECTLY; GRACEFULLY RAISE ARMS AND BEND ELBOWS. BRING HANDS IN TO TOUCH CHEST.

2. MOVE ARMS OUT AND STRAIGHT BACK AS FAR AS POSSIBLE. CLASP HANDS AND STRAIGHTEN ARMS.

3. GENTLY BEND BACKWARD FROM WAIST AS FAR AS POSSIBLE WITHOUT STRAIN, AND HOLD.

4. BRING CLASPED ARMS UP OVER BACK AND BEND FORWARD FROM WAIST AS FAR AS POSSIBLE. RELAX NECK AND HOLD.

5. *SLOWLY* STRAIGHTEN UP. UNCLASP HANDS. RELAX — REPEAT.

CHEST EXPANSION

You can expect to:

Develop the CHEST and BUST.

Firm and remove excess weight in the UPPER ARMS.

Improve the POSTURE.

Remove tension throughout the ENTIRE BODY.

Bring an increased supply of blood to the HEAD and BRAIN.

4. THE COMPLETE BREATH

This exercise can also be done sitting or lying without executing the arm movements. Perform 3 to 10 times.

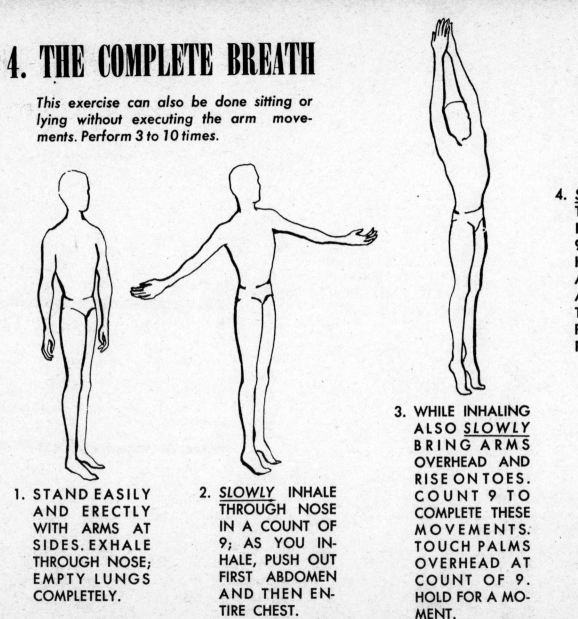

1. STAND EASILY AND ERECTLY WITH ARMS AT SIDES. EXHALE THROUGH NOSE; EMPTY LUNGS COMPLETELY.

2. *SLOWLY* INHALE THROUGH NOSE IN A COUNT OF 9; AS YOU INHALE, PUSH OUT FIRST ABDOMEN AND THEN ENTIRE CHEST.

3. WHILE INHALING ALSO *SLOWLY* BRING ARMS OVERHEAD AND RISE ON TOES. COUNT 9 TO COMPLETE THESE MOVEMENTS. TOUCH PALMS OVERHEAD AT COUNT OF 9. HOLD FOR A MOMENT.

4. *SLOWLY* EXHALE THROUGH NOSE IN A COUNT OF 9; AS YOU EXHALE, LOWER ARMS *SLOWLY* AND RETURN FEET TO FLOOR. REPEAT WITHOUT PAUSE.

THE COMPLETE BREATH

This exercise has a most positive effect on the entire organism in every one of its functions. Some specific results are:

Purification of the BLOOD resulting in a healthy and glowing SKIN and COMPLEXION.

Overcoming fatigue and regaining VITALITY.

Improvement in ALERTNESS and CLARITY OF MIND.

When you rise on your toes you strengthen the TOES, FEET, ANKLES and LEGS.

Through rising on your toes you also gain GRACE, BALANCE and POISE.

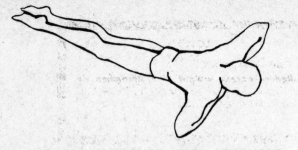

5. COBRA

1. LIE ON ABDOMEN; REST FOREHEAD ON FLOOR AND PLACE HANDS BENEATH SHOULDERS (FINGERS POINTING TOWARD ONE ANOTHER).

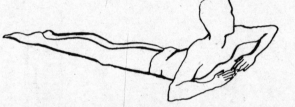

2. *SLOWLY* TILT HEAD BACKWARD AND BEGIN TO RAISE TRUNK BY PUSHING DOWN WITH HANDS.

COBRA

You can expect to:

Develop the CHEST and BUST.

Firm and strengthen the ARMS and BUTTOCKS.

Remove tension and stiffness throughout the NECK and BACK.

3. *SLOWLY* ARCH SPINE AND CONTINUE TO BRING TRUNK UP AND BACK AS FAR AS POSSIBLE WITHOUT STRAIN. HOLD YOUR EXTREME POSITION.

4. LOWER TRUNK IN THE EXACT REVERSE MOVEMENT, KEEPING THE SPINE ARCHED. REST CHEEK ON FLOOR. PLACE ARMS AT SIDES. RELAX— REPEAT.

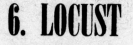

6. LOCUST

Count 5 to Raise; Hold 5; Lower 5; —
Perform 3 to 10 Times Alternating Legs

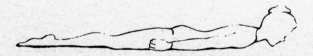

1. LIE ON ABDOMEN; REST CHIN ON FLOOR; MAKE TWO FISTS AND PLACE THEM NEAR SIDES.

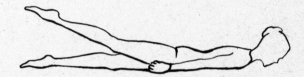

2. PUSH DOWN WITH FISTS AND RAISE RIGHT LEG _SLOWLY_ AS HIGH AS POSSIBLE. HOLD. KEEP KNEES STRAIGHT. KEEP CHIN ON FLOOR.

3. _SLOWLY_ LOWER RIGHT LEG.

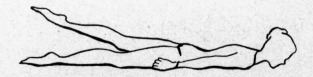

4. REPEAT MOVEMENTS WITH LEFT LEG.

7. LOTUS

Use the Lotus Posture to relax, breathe and meditate. Hold only as long as comfortable, then stretch legs straight out and gently massage knees.

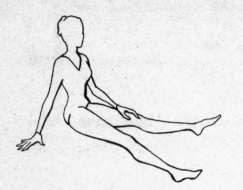

1. SIT WITH LEGS STRAIGHT OUT BEFORE YOU.

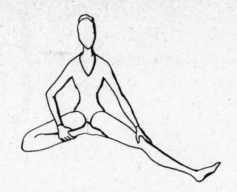

2. PLACE RIGHT FOOT SO THAT IT RESTS AGAINST THE UPPER PART OF THE LEFT THIGH.

> **LOTUS**
>
> **You can expect to:**
>
> Remove stiffness and loosen the FEET, ANKLES and KNEES.
>
> Reduce flabbiness and firm the THIGHS.
>
> Provides a comfortable sitting position for RELAXATION and MEDITATION.

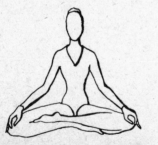

3. PLACE LEFT FOOT SO THAT IT IS IN THE FOLD OF RIGHT LEG. REST HANDS ON KNEES OR ON FLOOR BEHIND YOU. RELAX IN THIS POSITION FOR SEVERAL MINUTES.

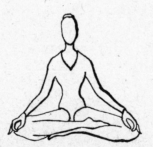

4. REVERSE THE LEGS.

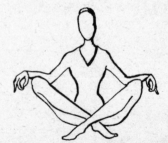

5. IF THIS POSTURE IS TOO DIFFICULT FOR YOU, SIT IN A SIMPLE CROSS-LEGGED POSTURE.

8. ABDOMINAL MOVEMENTS

Make sure movements are very rhythmical.
Do not rush. Perform 30-70 movements.

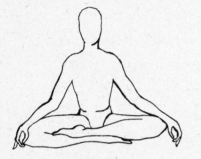

1. SIT IN THE LOTUS OR CROSS-LEGGED POSITION. REST HANDS ON KNEES OR ON FLOOR BEHIND YOU.

2. USE ABDOMINAL MUSCLES TO CONTRACT ABDOMEN AS FAR AS POSSIBLE AND HOLD FOR A SECOND.

3. ATTEMPT TO 'SNAP' ABDOMEN OUT IN A FORCEFUL MOVEMENT. REPEAT WITHOUT PAUSE. PERFORM 10 TIMES AND REST. REPEAT IN GROUPS OF 10.

9. ALTERNATE LEG PULLS

COUNT 30 SECONDS IN EXTREME PO-
SITION. PERFORM 3 TIMES EACH LEG.

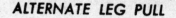
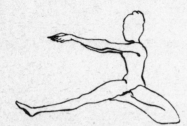

1. SIT WITH LEGS STRAIGHT
OUT BEFORE YOU. PLACE
LEFT FOOT AGAINST UPPER
INSIDE OF RIGHT THIGH.
SLOWLY AND *GRACEFULLY*
RAISE ARMS.

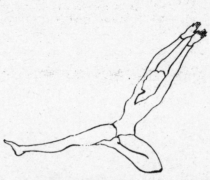

2. SLOWLY BRING ARMS UP
AND BACK AND LEAN
BACKWARD AS FAR AS
POSSIBLE.

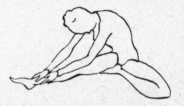

3. SLOWLY COME FORWARD
AND TAKE HOLD OF WHAT-
EVER PART OF RIGHT LEG
YOU CAN HOLD WITHOUT
STRAIN.

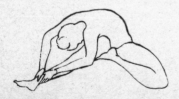

4. BEND ELBOWS OUTWARD
AND PULL TRUNK *SLOWLY*
DOWNWARD AS FAR AS
YOU CAN WITHOUT
STRAIN. HOLD WITHOUT
MOVEMENT.

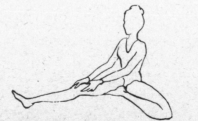

5. RELEASE LEG AND *SLOWLY*
STRAIGHTEN UP. REPEAT.

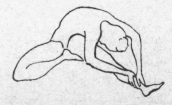

6. PERFORM IDENTICAL MOVE-
MENTS WITH LEFT LEG.

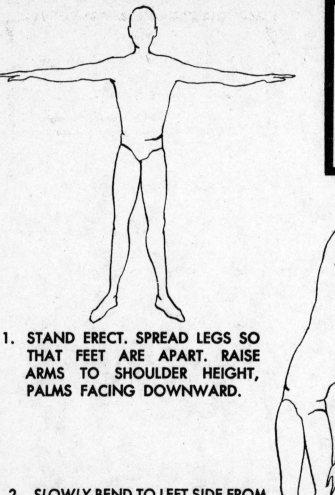

COUNT 5 FOR ALL MOVEMENTS—PERFORM 3 TIMES, ALTERNATING SIDES.

SIDE BEND

You can expect to: accomplish the following in the WAIST and HIPS; relieve tightness, reduce excess weight, overcome flabbiness and firm.

---

1. STAND ERECT. SPREAD LEGS SO THAT FEET ARE APART. RAISE ARMS TO SHOULDER HEIGHT, PALMS FACING DOWNWARD.

2. *SLOWLY BEND TO LEFT SIDE FROM WAIST; KEEP KNEES STRAIGHT; BRING RIGHT ARM OVERHEAD; ATTEMPT TO HAVE LEFT HAND TOUCH LEFT KNEE OR THIGH; ALLOW NECK TO GO LIMP.*

3. *SLOWLY STRAIGHTEN UP.*

4. PERFORM IDENTICAL MOVEMENTS TO THE RIGHT.

11. ROLL-TWIST

COUNT 3 IN EACH OF THE EXTREME PO-
SITIONS — PERFORM 4 TIMES CLOCKWISE;
4 TIMES COUNTER-CLOCKWISE.

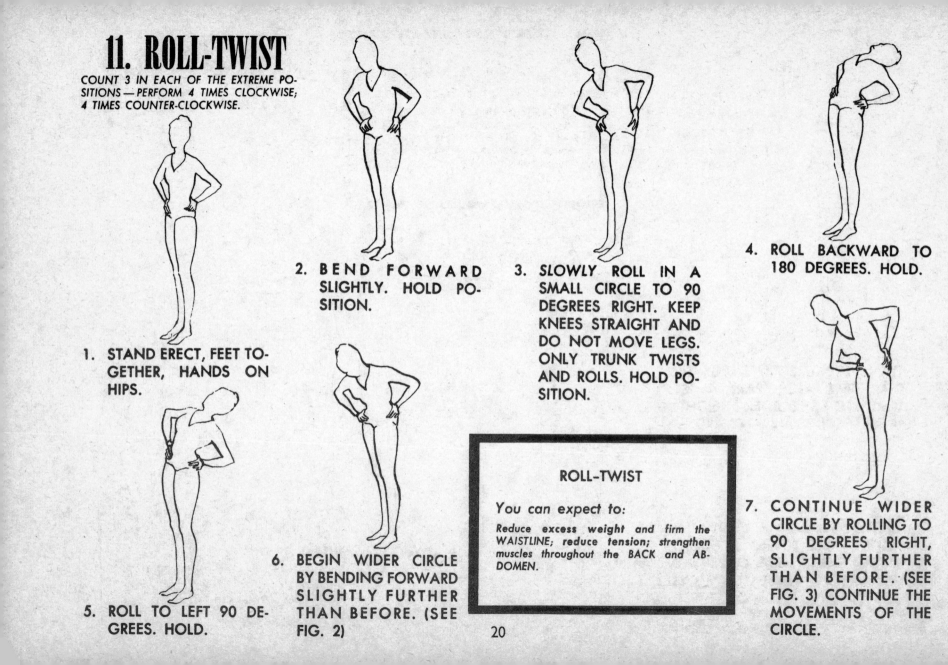

1. STAND ERECT, FEET TO-
GETHER, HANDS ON
HIPS.

2. BEND FORWARD
SLIGHTLY. HOLD PO-
SITION.

3. SLOWLY ROLL IN A
SMALL CIRCLE TO 90
DEGREES RIGHT. KEEP
KNEES STRAIGHT AND
DO NOT MOVE LEGS.
ONLY TRUNK TWISTS
AND ROLLS. HOLD PO-
SITION.

4. ROLL BACKWARD TO
180 DEGREES. HOLD.

5. ROLL TO LEFT 90 DE-
GREES. HOLD.

6. BEGIN WIDER CIRCLE
BY BENDING FORWARD
SLIGHTLY FURTHER
THAN BEFORE. (SEE
FIG. 2)

ROLL-TWIST

You can expect to:

*Reduce excess weight and firm the
WAISTLINE; reduce tension; strengthen
muscles throughout the BACK and AB-
DOMEN.*

7. CONTINUE WIDER
CIRCLE BY ROLLING TO
90 DEGREES RIGHT,
SLIGHTLY FURTHER
THAN BEFORE. (SEE
FIG. 3) CONTINUE THE
MOVEMENTS OF THE
CIRCLE.

Comments: Maintaining balance on the toes is difficult at first but as you continue to practice you will succeed. Then practice twisting on the toes to both sides. Never become discouraged and never laugh at yourself if you lose your balance. Come right back up at the point where the balance was lost and continue the exercise.

.COUNT 10 TO TWIST; HOLD EXTREME POSITION FOR 10; RETURN FRONTWARD IN 10 — PERFORM 2 TIMES EACH SIDE.

2. SLOWLY TWIST ARMS AND TRUNK 90 DEGREES TO THE LEFT; KEEP GAZE ON BACK OF HANDS; DO NOT MOVE LEGS. HOLD EXTREME POSITION.

1. STAND ERECT, FEET TOGETHER. *SLOWLY RAISE ARMS TO* SHOULDER LEVEL; LOOK AT BACK OF HANDS.

3. SLOWLY RETURN TO THE FRONTWARD POSITION.

STANDING—TWIST

You can expect to:

Reduce excess weight in the WAISTLINE; gain flexibility throughout the SPINE; regain youthful GRACE, BALANCE and POISE.

4. RISE ON TOES AND ATTEMPT TO TWIST IN INDENTICAL MANNER 90 DEGREES TO THE RIGHT. HOLD EXTREME POSITION. RETURN TO FRONTWARD POSITION, STILL ON TOES. LOWER LEGS AND ARMS. RELAX; REPEAT.

13. ARM & LEG STRETCH

COUNT 10 IN EXTREME POSITION —.PERFORM 3 TIMES EACH SIDE.

Comments: Practice to perform exercise without support of wall.

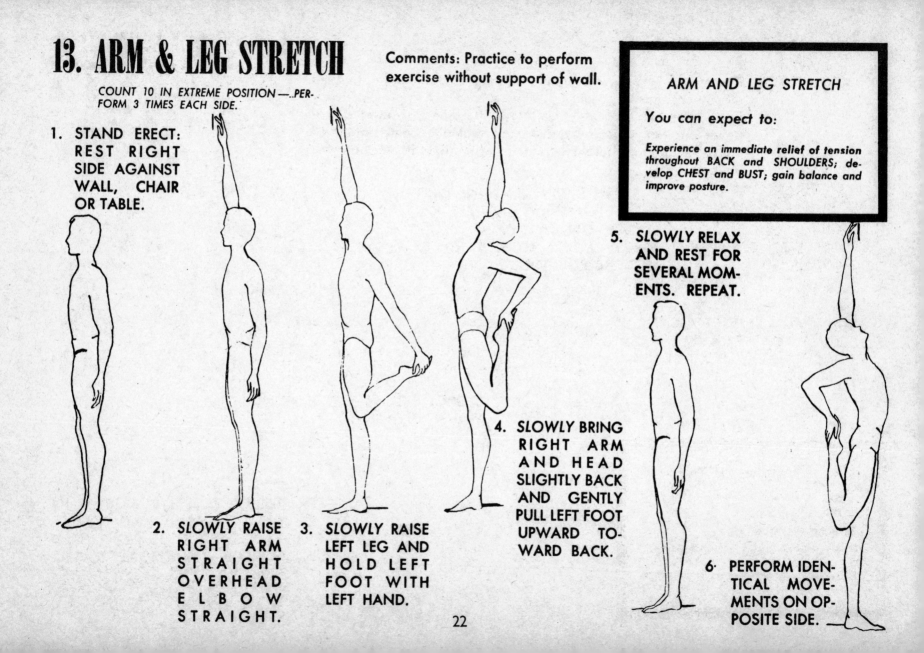

1. **STAND ERECT: REST RIGHT SIDE AGAINST WALL, CHAIR OR TABLE.**

2. *SLOWLY RAISE RIGHT ARM STRAIGHT OVERHEAD ELBOW STRAIGHT.*

3. *SLOWLY RAISE LEFT LEG AND HOLD LEFT FOOT WITH LEFT HAND.*

4. *SLOWLY BRING RIGHT ARM AND HEAD SLIGHTLY BACK AND GENTLY PULL LEFT FOOT UPWARD TOWARD BACK.*

5. *SLOWLY RELAX AND REST FOR SEVERAL MOMENTS. REPEAT.*

6. *PERFORM IDENTICAL MOVEMENTS ON OPPOSITE SIDE.*

ARM AND LEG STRETCH

You can expect to:

Experience an immediate relief of tension throughout BACK and SHOULDERS; develop CHEST and BUST; gain balance and improve posture.

22

14. LION

COUNT 30 TO 60 SECONDS IN EXTREME
POSITION — PERFORM 3 TO 5 TIMES.

Comments: Tongue must be extended as far as possible and with force for full benefits.

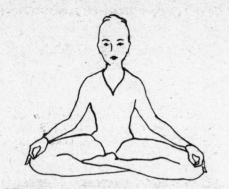

1. RELAX IN LOTUS OR CROSS-LEGGED POSTURE. REST HANDS ON KNEES.

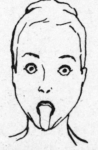

2. SPREAD FINGERS WIDE APART; LEAN FORWARD SLIGHTLY; WIDEN EYES; EXTEND TONGUE OUT AND DOWN WITH FORCE AND HOLD.

LION

You can expect to:

Firm and strengthen muscles throughout FACE and NECK; help prevent wrinkles and sagging; improve circulation and complexion.

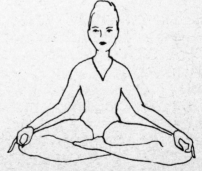

3. *VERY SLOWLY WITHDRAW TONGUE; RELAX EYES AND FINGERS. REPEAT.*

15. NECK MOVEMENTS

COUNT 20 TO 40 SECONDS FOR EACH OF THE 3 EXTREME POSITIONS — PERFORM 2 TO 3 TIMES.

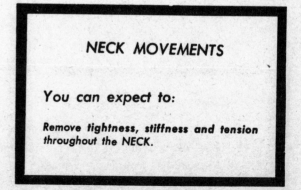

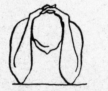

1. PLACE YOUR ELBOWS ON A LEVEL SURFACE (FLOOR, TABLE, DESK, ETC.) ELBOWS SHOULD BE FAIRLY CLOSE TOGETHER. CLASP HANDS ON LOWER BACK OF HEAD JUST ABOVE NECK AND GENTLY PUSH DOWN UNTIL CHIN RESTS AGAINST TOP OF CHEST. CLOSE EYES. DO NOT STRAIN. HOLD EXTREME POSITION. RELEASE SLOWLY.

2. DO NOT MOVE ARMS. TURN HEAD *SLOWLY* AND REST CHIN IN RIGHT PALM; REST LEFT HAND FIRMLY AGAINST BACK OF HEAD. TURN HEAD *SLOWLY* WITH HANDS AS FAR AS POSSIBLE TO RIGHT WITHOUT STRAIN. KEEP EYES CLOSED. HOLD EXTREME POSITION. RETURN *SLOWLY*.

3. DO NOT MOVE ARMS. TURN HEAD *SLOWLY* AND REST CHIN IN LEFT PALM: REST RIGHT HAND FIRMLY AGAINST BACK OF HEAD. TURN HEAD *SLOWLY* WITH HANDS AS FAR AS POSSIBLE TO LEFT WITHOUT STRAIN. KEEP EYES CLOSED. HOLD EXTREME POSITION. RETURN *SLOWLY*. REPEAT MOVEMENTS.

NECK MOVEMENTS

You can expect to:

Remove tightness, stiffness and tension throughout the NECK.

Comments: Head is not to be moved quickly, jerked or forced.

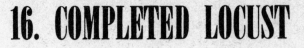

Comments: The muscles needed to perform this exercise correctly and gain the wonderful benefits, will become strengthened through simple repetition. Do not be discouraged if you find these muscles weak during early attempts.

COUNT 5 TO RAISE LEGS; HOLD 5; LOWER 5 — PERFORM 3 TIMES.

COMPLETED LOCUST (FOR PRELIMIN-INARY LOCUST SEE EXERCISE 6)

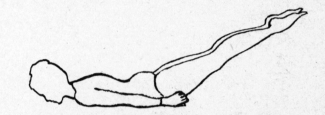

1. LIE ON ABDOMEN; REST CHIN ON FLOOR; MAKE TWO FISTS OUT OF HANDS AND PLACE THUMB DOWNWARD NEAR SIDES.

2. PUSH DOWN HARD WITH FISTS AND ATTEMPT TO RAISE BOTH LEGS FROM THE FLOOR; KEEP KNEES STRAIGHT; KEEP CHIN ON FLOOR AND DO NOT RAISE HEAD. HOLD EXTREME POSITION.

COMPLETED LOCUST

You can expect to:

Reduce excess weight and greatly strengthen, develop and streamline the LEGS, THIGHS, HIPS AND BUTTOCKS.

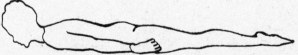

3. SLOWLY LOWER LEGS; REST CHEEK ON FLOOR. RELAX UNTIL READY TO REPEAT.

17. BOW

COUNT 10 TO 20 SECONDS IN EXTREME POSITION — PERFORM 3 TIMES.

Comments: It may be necessary to perform only the preliminary bow in the beginning. Gradually the muscles necessary to raise the knees will be developed through practice of the Locust.

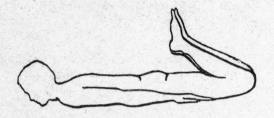

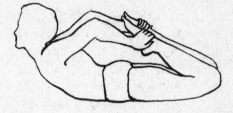

1. LIE ON ABDOMEN: REST ARMS AT SIDES AND CHIN ON FLOOR: BEND LEGS AT KNEES AND BRING HEELS IN.

2. REACH BACK AND ATTEMPT TO HOLD BOTH FEET WITH HANDS.

3. HOLD YOUR FEET FIRMLY AND *SLOWLY* AND *EASILY* RAISE YOUR TRUNK FROM THE FLOOR, HOLDING HEAD BACK. HOLD. THIS IS THE PRELIMINARY BOW.

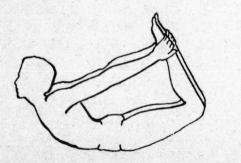

BOW

You can expect to:
Greatly strengthen and develop the entire SPINE, particularly in the LUMBAR area; develop CHEST and BUST and improve POSTURE.

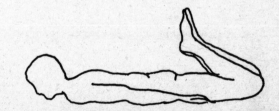

4. KEEPING THE TRUNK RAISED, ATTEMPT NOW TO BRING THE KNEES UP. KEEP THE KNEES AS CLOSE TOGETHER AS POSSIBLE. HOLD EXTREME POSITION.

5. SLOWLY LOWER KNEES AND CHIN TO FLOOR; RELEASE FEET AND SLOWLY LOWER LEGS TO FLOOR.

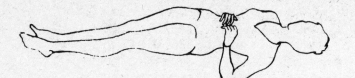

18. DIRECTING THE LIFE FORCE

1. LIE ON BACK, EYES CLOSED. REST FINGERTIPS OF BOTH HANDS ON SOLAR PLEXUS. *SLOWLY INHALE AND VISUALIZE A WHITE LIGHT BEING DRAWN FROM SOLAR PLEXUS INTO FINGERTIPS.*

COUNT 10 FOR INHALATION; COUNT 3 TO TRANSFER FINGERTIPS; COUNT 10 FOR EXHALATION — PERFORM A MINIMUM 10-25 TIMES. REPEAT AS OFTEN DURING DAY AS REQUIRED.

Comments: To receive the most effective aid from this exercise you must concentrate carefully on the movements and attempt always to visualize the light. This ability to visualize will come easily with practice.

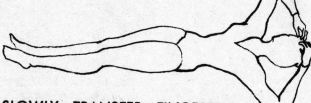

2. SLOWLY TRANSFER FINGERTIPS TO FOREHEAD AND EXHALE, VISUALIZING WHITE LIGHT FLOWING INTO HEAD.

3. RETURN FINGERTIPS TO SOLAR PLEXUS AND REPEAT.

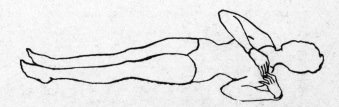

DIRECTING THE LIFE FORCE

You can expect to:

Gain TRANQUILITY and CALMNESS by directing energy from the SOLAR PLEXUS throughout the HEAD or to wherever it is needed.

4. DURING EXHALATION, FINGERTIPS MAY BE DIRECTED TO ANY PART OF THE BODY TO AID IN RELIEF OF TENSION, PAIN OR DISCOMFORT.

19. SHOULDER STAND

BEGIN WITH 30 SECONDS IN YOUR EXTREME POSITION AND GRADUALLY EXTEND TIME UNTIL YOU CAN HOLD FROM 3 TO 5 MINUTES.

1. LIE ON BACK, ARMS AT SIDES; ALLOW BODY TO GO COMPLETELY LIMP.

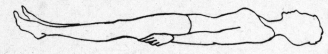

2. TURN PALMS DOWNWARD; STIFFEN LEG AND ABDOMINAL MUSCLES AND SLOWLY RAISE LEGS WITH KNEES STRAIGHT TO RIGHT ANGLE POSITION.

3. PUSH DOWN HARD WITH PALMS AND ATTEMPT TO RAISE WAIST AND HIPS FROM FLOOR.

4. PROP HANDS AGAINST WAIST OR BACK AND SLOWLY STRAIGHTEN UP. STOP AND HOLD AT WHATEVER POINT YOU ARE ABLE TO REACH.

5. IF POSSIBLE, STRAIGHTEN TO EXTREME VERTICAL POSITION AND HOLD. CLOSE EYES AND CONCENTRATE ON SLOW, RHYTHMIC BREATHING.

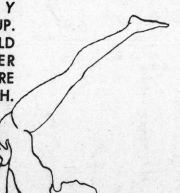

SHOULDER STAND

You can expect to:

Stimulate the THYROID GLAND as an aid to weight normalizing and control; improve BLOOD CIRCULATION in upper areas of the body; refresh and stimulate numerous ORGANS and GLANDS through the inversion; relax LEGS and often help VEIN and ARTERY conditions.

28

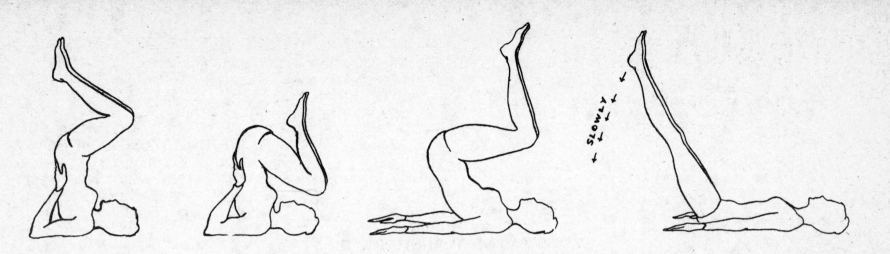

6. **BEND KNEES AND** *SLOWLY* **LOWER KNEES TOWARD HEAD.**

7. **LOWER KNEES UNTIL KNEES ARE BROUGHT DOWN AS FAR AS POSSIBLE.**

8. **PLACE HANDS BACK ON FLOOR AND ROLL FORWARD** *SLOWLY* **AND WITH CONTROL, ARCHING NECK BACKWARD AS YOU ROLL FORWARD TO** *PREVENT HEAD FROM LEAVING FLOOR.*

9. **WHEN WAIST AND HIPS REST ON FLOOR, STRAIGHTEN LEGS STRAIGHT UP AND** *VERY SLOWLY* **LOWER TO FLOOR.**

Comments: Any angle of inversion is better than none. Go up as far as you can and simply hold your extreme position. Gradually you will be able to straighten further. If you cannot bring your waist from the floor in the beginning, you can roll back quickly with your legs giving you enough momentum to leave the floor. As an alternate method. you can place your legs against the wall and walk up the wall until you achieve any angle of inversion. If you have a heart condition or high blood pressure, it is best, as always, to consult your physician before attempting the shoulder stand.

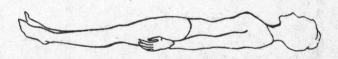

10. **ALLOW BODY TO GO COMPLETELY LIMP.**

20. PLOUGH

BEGIN WITH 20 SECONDS IN YOUR EXTREME POSITION AND GRADUALLY EXTEND TIME TO 1 MINUTE — PERFORM 2-3 TIMES.

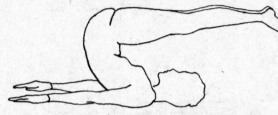

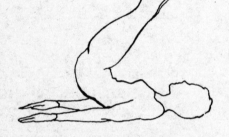

1. LIE ON YOUR BACK
   THE FIRST THREE MOVEMENTS ARE IDENTICAL WITH THE SHOULDER STAND.

PLOUGH

You can expect to:
Gain great strength and flexibility throughout the SPINE, BACK and NECK; improve blood circulation; develop and firm muscles of the ABDOMEN.

---

2. INSTEAD OF STRAIGHTENING THE TRUNK AS IN THE SHOULDER STAND, KEEP THE PALMS ON THE FLOOR AND CONTINUE TO BRING THE LEGS BACK AS FAR AS POSSIBLE. HOLD YOUR EXTREME POSITION. DO NOT BEND THE KNEES.

3. IF POSSIBLE, ALLOW THE FEET TO TOUCH THE FLOOR BEHIND YOU. THE KNEES MUST NOT BEND. HOLD THE POSITION WITHOUT MOVEMENT.

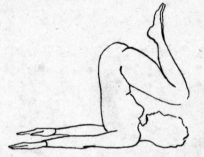

4. BEND THE KNEES AND BRING THEM TOWARD THE FOREHEAD. PROCEED FROM THIS POINT EXACTLY AS IN THE SHOULDER STAND UNTIL YOUR ENTIRE BODY IS RESTING ONCE AGAIN ON THE FLOOR.

Comments: There is no hurry to reach the extreme posture as in Fig.3. Go only as far as you can, keeping your knees straight and hold your extreme position. Do not strain. Gradually your legs will lower to the floor.

21. HIP BEND

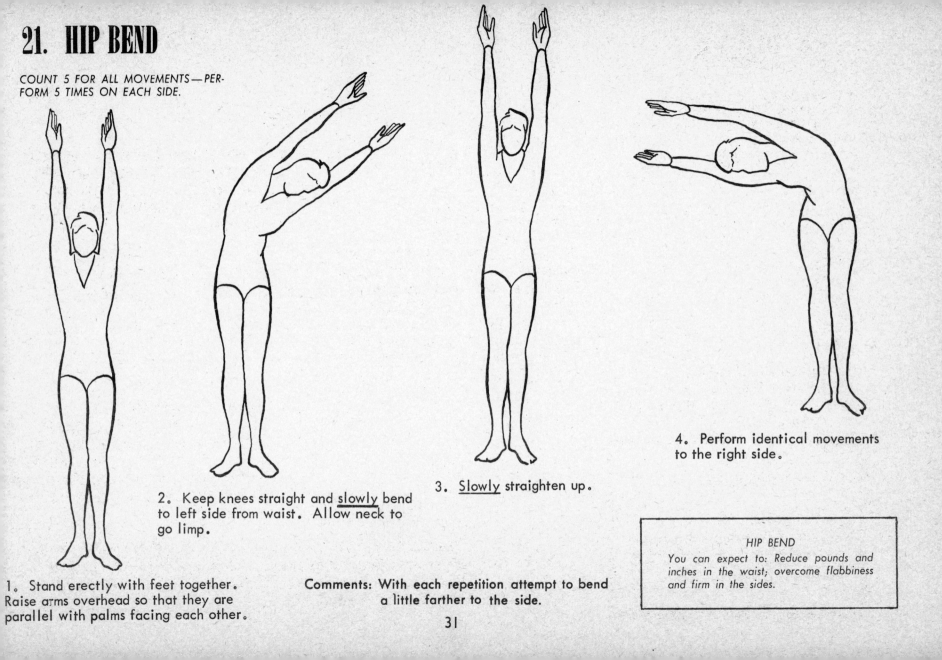

1. Stand erectly with feet together.
Raise arms overhead so that they are
parallel with **palms facing each other.**

2. Keep knees straight and <u>slowly</u> bend
to left side from waist. Allow neck to
go limp.

3. <u>Slowly</u> straighten up.

4. Perform identical movements
to the right side.

Comments: With each repetition attempt to bend
a little farther to the side.

HIP BEND
*You can expect to: Reduce pounds and
inches in the waist; overcome flabbiness
and firm in the sides.*

31

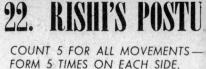

COUNT 5 FOR ALL MOVEMENTS—
FORM 5 TIMES ON EACH SIDE.

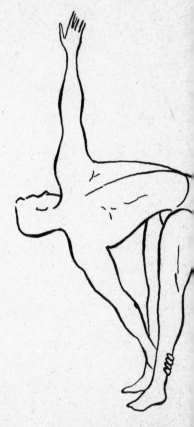

1. Stand erect with feet slightly apart and raise arms as illustrated.

2. Bend slowly at the waist so that the right hand slides down the back of the right leg and the eyes look at the left hand. Keep the knees straight.

3. Slowly straighten up bringing arms into position illustrated.

4. Repeat on opposite si

Comments: Attempt to bend a little farther with each repetition. Remember to turn your head so that your eyes can always see the back of your hand in the extreme position.

RISHI'S POSTURE
You can expect to: Promote flexibility; streamline the entire body; gain balance, grace and poise.

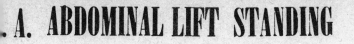

.A. ABDOMINAL LIFT STANDING

PERFORM 10 TIMES TO EACH EXHALA-
TION. DO 30-70 MOVEMENTS IN ALL.

Place body in squatting position
ustrated. Note carefully that the
es are slightly bent and hands
t on upper thighs, all fingers
ned inward.

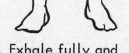

2. Exhale fully and
perform Abdominal Lift.

3. 'Snap' abdomen out in forceful
movement. Repeat rhythmically
10 times. Straighten up and rest.

ABDOMINAL LIFTS

*You can expect to: Reduce excess weight
and firm the entire abdomen; stimulate organs and glands of the viscera.*

PERFORM 10 TIMES TO EACH EXHALATION. DO 30-70 MOVEMENTS IN ALL.

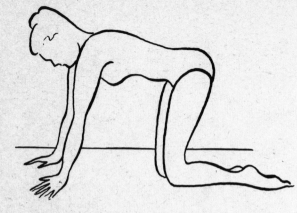

1. Place body in all fours position as illustrated.

Comments: Remember that the air is complete exhaled and held of the lungs during each group of 10 movements. not sacrifice rhythmic and forceful movements for spe

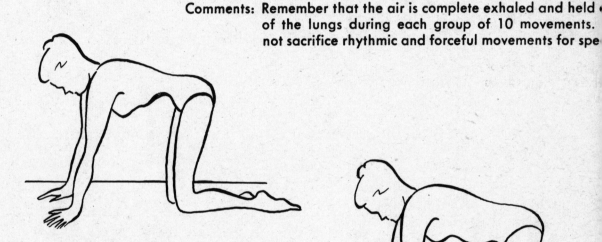

2. Exhale fully and perform Abdominal Lift.

3. 'Snap' abdomen out in forceful movement. Repeat rhythmically, without pause, 10 times. Sit back on heels and rest.
Repeat in groups of 10.

ABDOMINAL LIFTS
You can expect to: Reduce excess weight and firm the entire abdomen; stimulate organs and glands of the viscera.

---

4. SIMPLE TWIST

OUNT 5 IN EXTREME POSITION—
RFORM 3 TIMES EACH SIDE

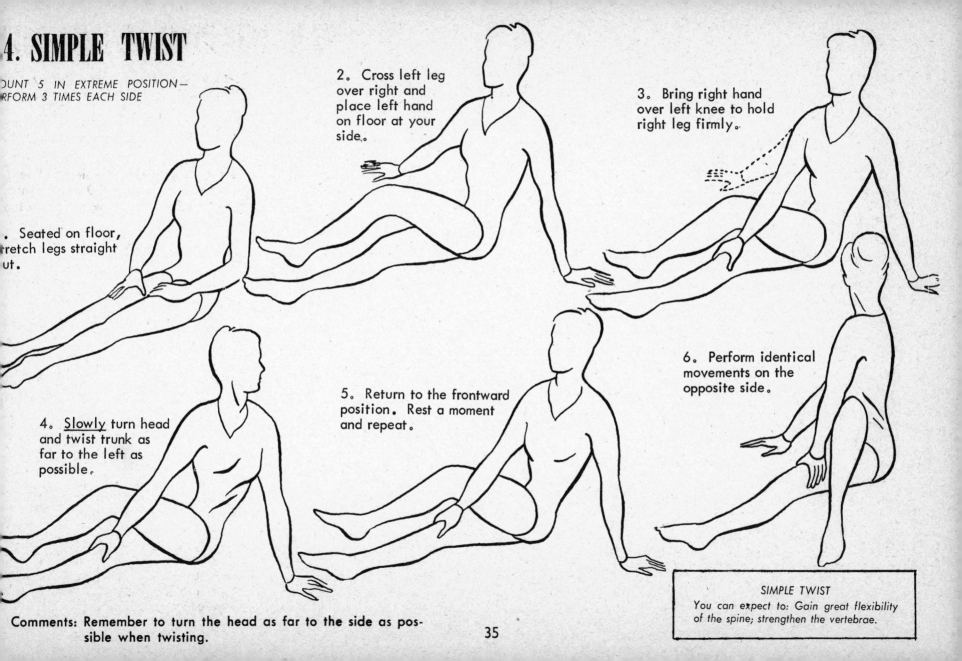

. Seated on floor, tretch legs straight ut.

2. Cross left leg over right and place left hand on floor at your side.

3. Bring right hand over left knee to hold right leg firmly.

4. Slowly turn head and twist trunk as far to the left as possible.

5. Return to the frontward position. Rest a moment and repeat.

6. Perform identical movements on the opposite side.

SIMPLE TWIST
You can expect to: Gain great flexibility of the spine; strengthen the vertebrae.

Comments: Remember to turn the head as far to the side as possible when twisting.

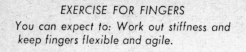

EXERCISE FOR FINGERS
You can expect to: Work out stiffness and keep fingers flexible and agile.

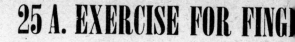

1. Grasp each finger of the right hand with the left hand and pull gently.

2. Perform the identical movements with fingers of the left hand.

EXERCISE FOR ELBOWS
You can expect to: Work out stiffness and tension in elbows.

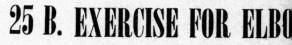

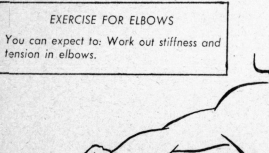

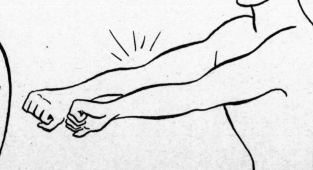

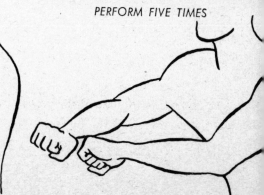

1. Bring arms into position illustrated (Elbows bent).

2. 'Snap' arms straight out to exercise elbows.

3. Return arms to sta position and repeat.

6. EYE EXERCISE

OP MOMENTARILY AT EACH POSI-
ON—PERFORM 10 TIMES CLOCKWISE;
TIMES COUNTER-CLOCKWISE.

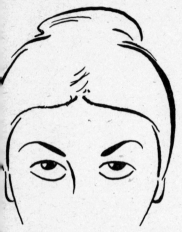

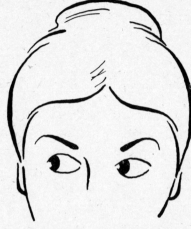

After 10 Repetitions, perform 10 identical
movements counter-clockwise.

1. Move eyes to extreme top
of socket. Hold one second.

2. Roll eyes to extreme right
and hold one second.

Comments: Only the eyes move. Do not move the head.

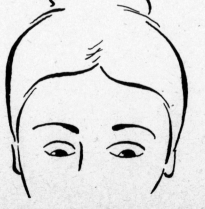

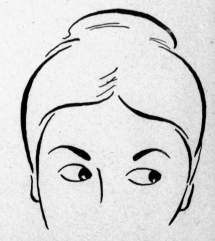

3. Roll eyes to extreme bottom
and hold one second.

4. Roll eyes to extreme left
and hold one second.

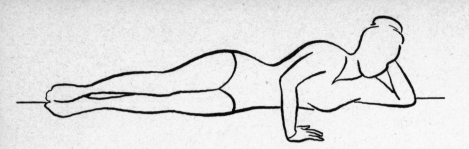

1. Place body in position illustrated.

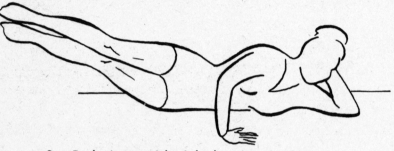

SIDE RAISE

You can expect to: Firm and regain muscle tone throughout the legs, thighs, hips, buttocks.

2. Push down with right hand and raise legs as high as possible.

3. Lower legs <u>slowly</u> and relax for a few moments. Repeat.

Comments: Bring your legs up directly from the side without swaying off to the right or left. Push down hard with your hand to aid in the raise.

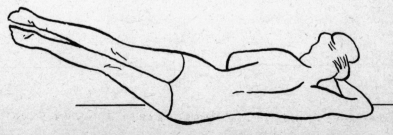

4. Perform identical movements on right side.

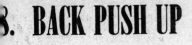

8. BACK PUSH UP

UNT 10 IN EXTREME POSITION—
FORM 5 TIMES.

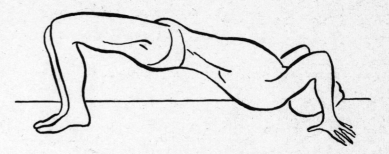

1. Place body in position illustrated.

2. Push down hard with hands and feet and raise body as high as possible. Hold.

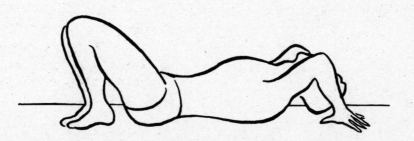

3. Lower body <u>slowly</u> and relax. Repeat.

Comments: Arch neck slightly as you raise. This enables you to get up higher.

BACK PUSH UP

You can expect to: Firm and maintain muscle tone throughout the legs, thighs, buttocks and upper arms.

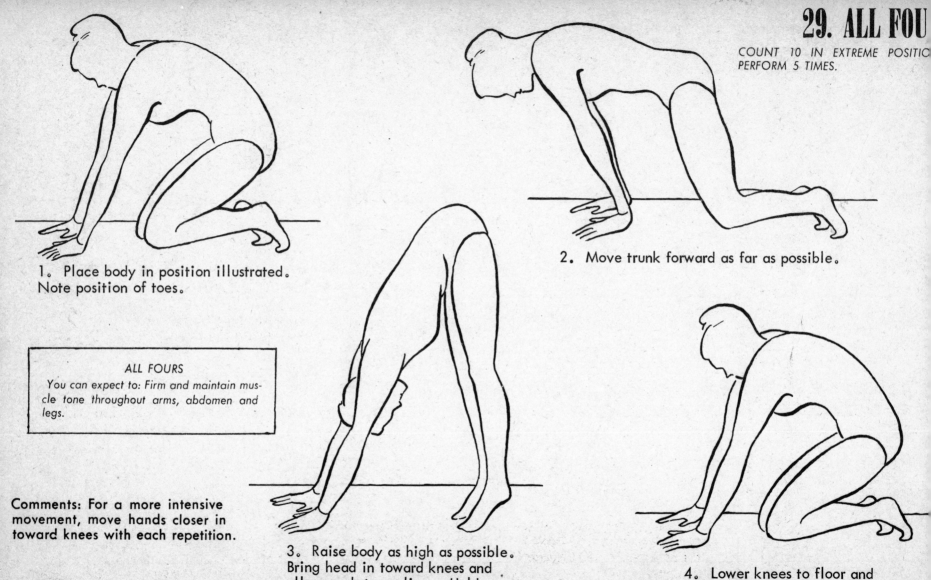

1. Place body in position illustrated.
Note position of toes.

2. Move trunk forward as far as possible.

ALL FOURS
You can expect to: Firm and maintain muscle tone throughout arms, abdomen and legs.

Comments: For a more intensive movement, move hands closer in toward knees with each repetition.

3. Raise body as high as possible.
Bring head in toward knees and allow neck to go limp. Hold.

4. Lower knees to floor and sit on heels. Repeat.

O. LEG CLASP

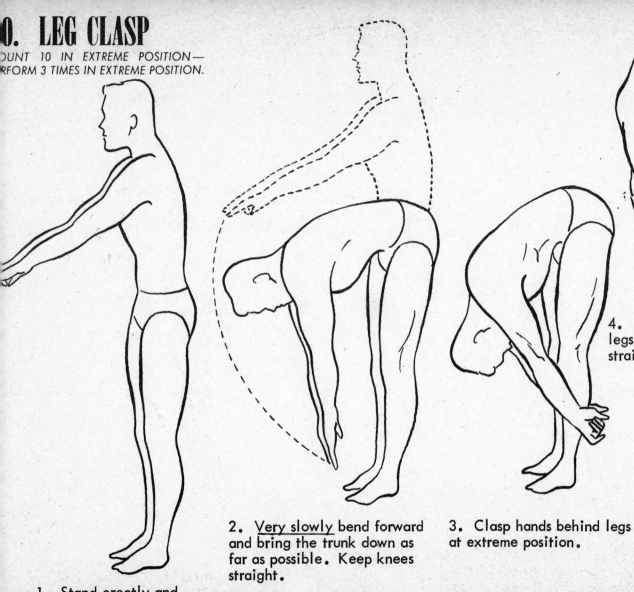

4. Pull trunk as far toward legs as possible without strain. Hold.

5. Relax the stretch but keep hands clasped as illustrated. Perform 3 times. Unclasp hands and straighten up <u>very slowly</u>.

2. <u>Very slowly</u> bend forward and bring the trunk down as far as possible. Keep knees straight.

3. Clasp hands behind legs at extreme position.

1. Stand erectly and extend arms as illustrated.

LEG CLASP

You can expect to: Gain great flexibility of the spine; stretch and strengthen the muscles and ligaments of the legs.

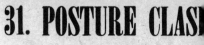

COUNT 5 IN EXTREME POSITION —
FORM 5 MOVEMENTS UP AND 5 MO
MENTS DOWN ON EACH SIDE.

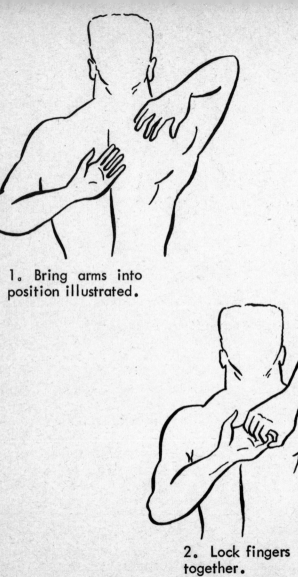

1. Bring arms into
position illustrated.

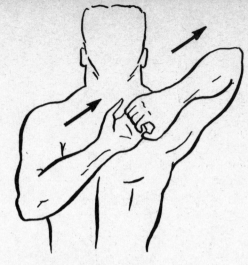

3. Pull gently with
the right arm. Hold.

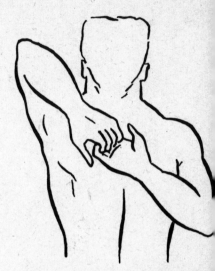

5. Repeat on opposite side

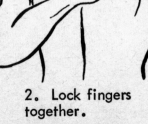

2. Lock fingers
together.

4. Pull down gently
with left arm. Hold.

Comments: This exercise may be performed either sitting or standing. If the hands will not meet behind the back, use
handkerchief or piece of cloth and hold ends with hands.

2. FULL TWIST

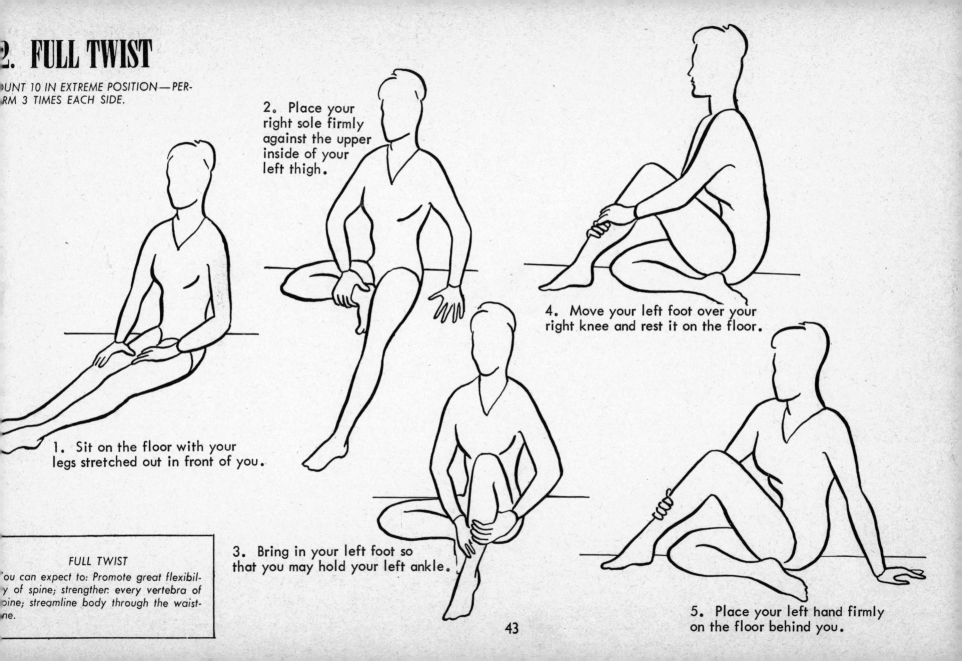

2. Place your right sole firmly against the upper inside of your left thigh.

4. Move your left foot over your right knee and rest it on the floor.

1. Sit on the floor with your legs stretched out in front of you.

3. Bring in your left foot so that you may hold your left ankle.

5. Place your left hand firmly on the floor behind you.

FULL TWIST

You can expect to: Promote great flexibil-
y of spine; strengthen every vertebra of
pine; streamline body through the waist-
ne.

43

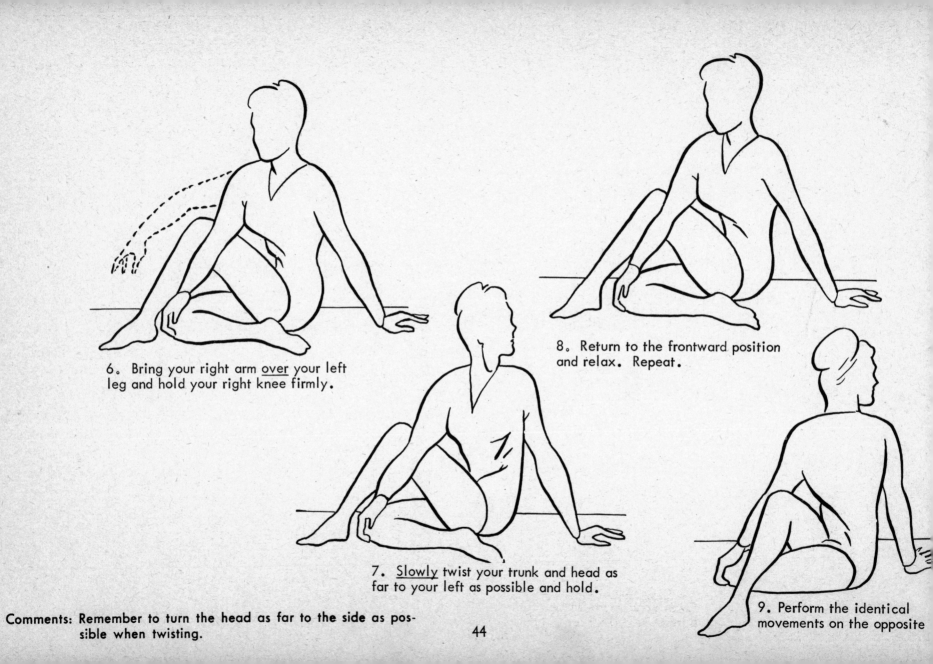

6. Bring your right arm <u>over</u> your left leg and hold your right knee firmly.

7. <u>Slowly</u> twist your trunk and head as far to your left as possible and hold.

8. Return to the frontward position and relax. Repeat.

9. Perform the identical movements on the opposite

Comments: Remember to turn the head as far to the side as possible when twisting.

33. OVERHEAD SQUAT

MOVEMENTS ARE DONE IN CONTINU-
OUS MOTION—PERFORM 5 TIMES.

1. Place hands with palms
together in position indicated.
(Hands do not touch head.)

2. Very slowly bend knees and
lower body until resting on heels.
(Note position of feet.)

3. Very slowly raise body
until standing on toes.

4. Lower body to position
1 and repeat.

STOP MOMENTARILY IN EACH
FOUR POSITIONS—PERFORM 5
CLOCKWISE; 5 TIMES COUNTER-
WISE.

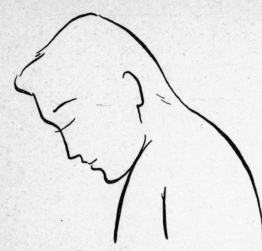

1. <u>Slowly</u> bend the head forward and
allow the chin to rest against the chest.

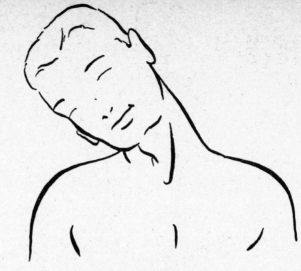

2. <u>Slowly</u> roll and twist
the head to the extreme right.

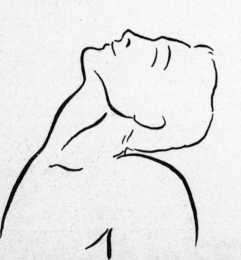

3. <u>Slowly</u> roll and twist the head
to the extreme backward position.
(Feel the chin and throat stretching.)

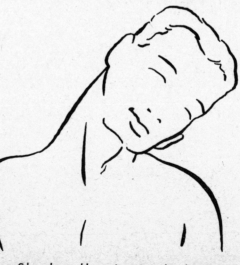

4. <u>Slowly</u> roll and twist the head
to the extreme left.

NECK ROLL
You can expect to: Relieve stiffness
tension in the neck.

46

KNEE & THIGH STRETCH

COUNT 10 IN EXTREME POSITION—PER-
FORM 5 TIMES.

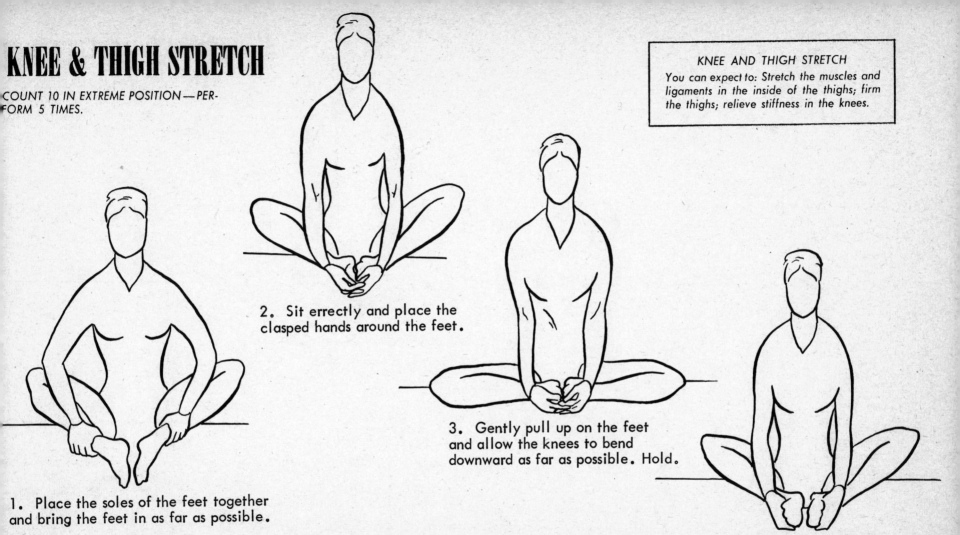

2. Sit errectly and place the clasped hands around the feet.

1. Place the soles of the feet together and bring the feet in as far as possible.

3. Gently pull up on the feet and allow the knees to bend downward as far as possible. Hold.

4. Relax and repeat.

Comments: Remember to remain sitting erectly throughout the exercise. Even if the knees move only a few inches in the beginning, this exercise will be of great benefit to you.

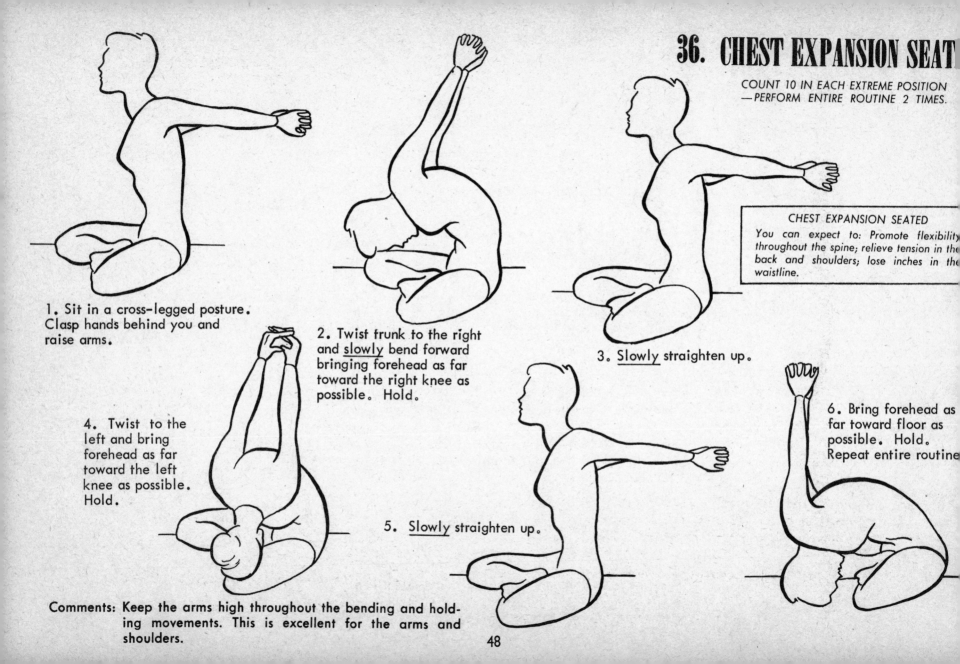

COUNT 10 IN EACH EXTREME POSITION
—PERFORM ENTIRE ROUTINE 2 TIMES.

CHEST EXPANSION SEATED

You can expect to: Promote flexibility throughout the spine; relieve tension in the back and shoulders; lose inches in the waistline.

---

1. Sit in a cross-legged posture. Clasp hands behind you and raise arms.

2. Twist trunk to the right and <u>slowly</u> bend forward bringing forehead as far toward the right knee as possible. Hold.

3. <u>Slowly</u> straighten up.

4. Twist to the left and bring forehead as far toward the left knee as possible. Hold.

5. <u>Slowly</u> straighten up.

6. Bring forehead as far toward floor as possible. Hold. Repeat entire routine

Comments: Keep the arms high throughout the bending and holding movements. This is excellent for the arms and shoulders.

SIT UP; LIE DOWN

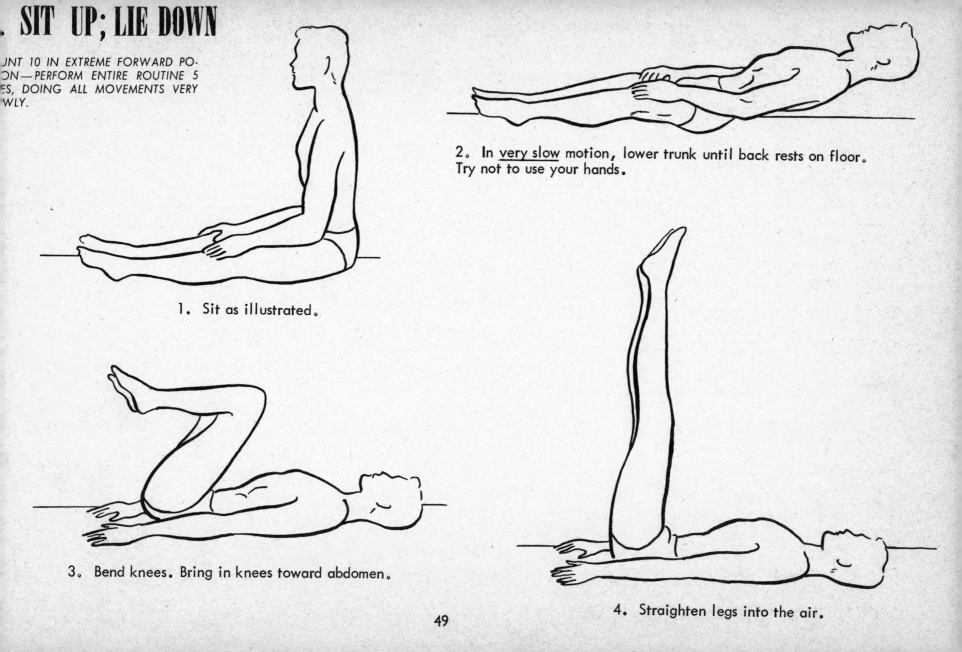

1. Sit as illustrated.

2. In <u>very slow</u> motion, lower trunk until back rests on floor. Try not to use your hands.

3. Bend knees. Bring in knees toward abdomen.

4. Straighten legs into the air.

Comments: Hold legs an inch from the floor in Position 5 for an extra few seconds for maximum toning.

6. Raise trunk <u>very slowly</u> without use of hands and from sitting position slowly slide hands as far down legs as possible. Hold.

5. <u>Very slowly</u>, lower legs to floor.

7. <u>Slowly</u> straighten up into fir position and repeat entire routi

LEG OVER

10 IN EXTREME POSITION—
ATE LEGS AND PERFORM 5 TIMES
DE.

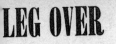

2. <u>Slowly</u> bring the leg over and down to touch floor if possible. Keep both shoulders on the floor. Hold.

1. In a lying position raise the right leg as illustrated.

> **LEG OVER**
> You can expect to: Streamline the waist and hips.

Comments: In the extreme position (Figs. 2 and 4) try to keep th
leg toward the head so that it makes a right angle wit
the body. Make sure both shoulders remain on the floo

3. Slowly bring the right leg back to the position
of Fig. 1 and slowly lower to the floor.

4. Repeat with the left leg.

39. HEAD STAND

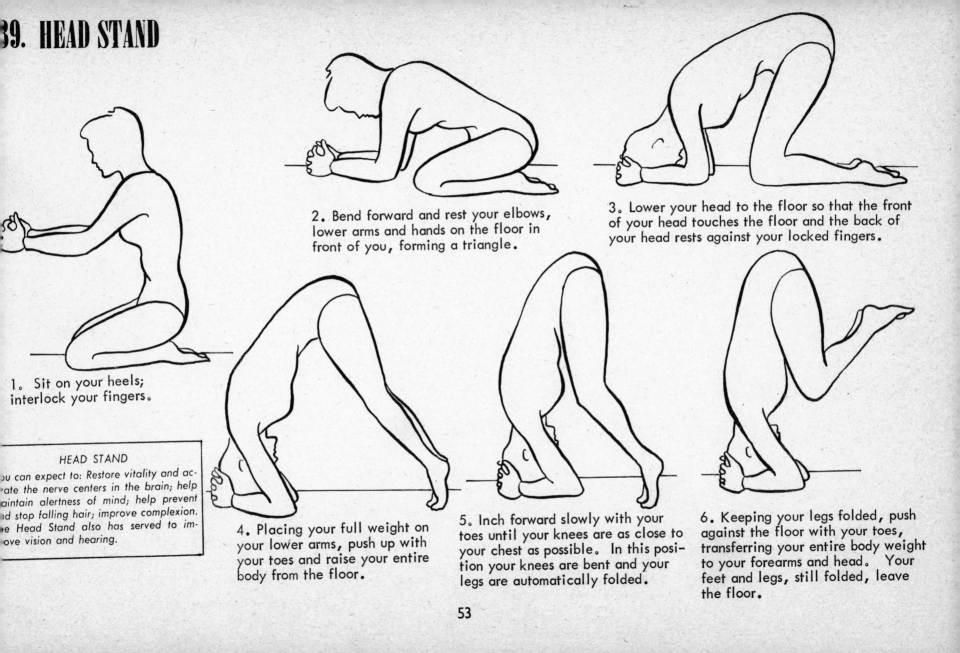

2. Bend forward and rest your elbows, lower arms and hands on the floor in front of you, forming a triangle.

3. Lower your head to the floor so that the front of your head touches the floor and the back of your head rests against your locked fingers.

1. Sit on your heels; interlock your fingers.

HEAD STAND

ou can expect to: Restore vitality and ac-
ate the nerve centers in the brain; help
aintain alertness of mind; help prevent
d stop falling hair; improve complexion.
e Head Stand also has served to im-
ove vision and hearing.

4. Placing your full weight on your lower arms, push up with your toes and raise your entire body from the floor.

5. Inch forward slowly with your toes until your knees are as close to your chest as possible. In this position your knees are bent and your legs are automatically folded.

6. Keeping your legs folded, push against the floor with your toes, transferring your entire body weight to your forearms and head. Your feet and legs, still folded, leave the floor.

The HEAD STAND (either Modified or Complete) *is done only once, beginning with 15 seconds and adding 15 seconds each week until you reach 3 minutes. When you are secure in the HEAD STAND you may want to remain in this position longer than 3 minutes which is perfectly feasible. Place your watch where you may glance at it as necessary.*

8. To do the Complete Head Stand continue from the position of step (7) by <u>slowly</u> straightening your knees and raising your legs, one inch at a time, until your body is in a vertical position. There is no hurry to accomplish the completed position.

7. Continue to place all your weight on your forearms and your head; raise your folded legs until the trunk is inverted. This is the Modified Head Stand and is as far as you should go at first. Do not try to straighten your legs until you have complete mastery of this posture.

If you are skeptical about being able to maintain your balance in the Head Stand, then use the wall for support. Place youself about 6 inches from the wall and you can balance yourself against it if your go too far forward in steps (6), (7) or (8). If you use the wall and you allow it to support your legs and back, continue to push yourself easily away from the wall with your feet and try to balance yourself. You can also use a pillow under your head to prevent any soreness. Make your surrounding area soft with a few pillows, blankets, etc. so that if you fall sidewise or forward you will be protected.

ALTERNATE NOSTRIL BREATHING

COUNT AS INDICATED — PERFORM 7
TIMES WITH EACH NOSTRIL.

ALTERNATE NOSTRIL BREATHING
You can expect to: Experience a natural
feeling of calmness and tranquility; clear
the breathing passages; help relieve head-
aches.

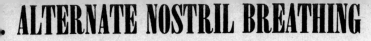

. Place the right hand
nd fingers as illustrated.

2. Press the right nostril closed with the
thumb and inhale <u>slowly</u> and quietly through
the left nostril in a count of 8 beats.

3. Close both nostrils and
retain the air for 8 beats.

4. Release the right nostril (still
holding the left closed) and exhale
<u>slowly</u> and quietly through the right
nostril in a count of 8 beats.

5. Keep the left nostril closed and without pause, inhale <u>slowly</u> and quietly through the right nostril
in a count of 8 beats. Close both nostrils and hold for 8. Release the left nostril (keeping the right
closed) and exhale <u>slowly</u> and quietly through the left nostril in a count of 8 beats. Repeat entire
routine 7 times.

Comments: Close the eyes. Keep the hand relaxed. Breathe quietly
and deeply. Repeat as often as necessary for a natural
tranquilizer.

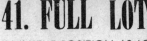

REMAIN IN THE POSITION AS LO...
IS COMFORTABLE.

1. Place the left foot as high on the right thigh as possible.

2. If the left knee can touch the floor without strain, you should be able to do the Full Lotus by placing the right foot on the left thigh. In the beginning hold the posture for a short time and try alternating the legs.

3. The classical Full Lotus meditation posture is accomplished by placing the hands and fingers in the position illustrated.

Comments:

The Full Lotus is an advanced posture. It is a difficult position for most people and one should not become discouraged if it does not come quickly. You can practice for the Full Lotus by practicing with Exercise 7 in the first book.

4. A variation with the Full Lotus is to place the hands on each side and raise the body. This is the Raised Lotus for strengthening and developing the arms and wrists. It is held a few seconds and repeated five times.

LIFETIME PLAN OF PRACTICE

The following chart presents a clear, simple and concise way for
u to practise every one of the wonderful Yoga exercises from the
OGA FOR HEALTH book in approximately 20-30 minutes per
y. The plan should be used as follows: The numbers 1, 2 and 3
 the top of the chart refer to 'days'. One of the three groups of
ercises are used on each practice day and they are used con-
utively. For example, on Monday you would practise Group 1,
 Tuesday, Group 2, on Wednesday, Group 3. Then on
ursday, you would return to Group 1, on Friday, Group 2, etc.
 is important that you keep note of which group you have done on
ch day because if your practice is interrupted for any reason, then
u should take up on the next practice day where you left off.
at is, if you were to practise Group 1 on Monday, Group 2 on
esday and you were unable to practise on Wednesday, then you
uld begin with Group 3 when you practised on Thursday. In this
nner you will include all of the exercises in each three days of
actice.

The time of the day when you practise is up to you. Fit your
actice into your schedule as best you can, but once you begin
 practise try not to be interrupted. It may be convenient for you
 practise half of the exercises in any one group in the morning
d then do the rest of that group later in the day. If you practise
th me during our television programme, then you use the chart
 practice later in the day or when you miss the programme. You
o use the chart for weekend and holiday practice

Remember that all of the information regarding the number
 repetitions and the time for holding in each of the exercises is
en to you just beneath the name of the exercise in the book.

You should follow this information closely until you become quite
adept with the exercises. Then you can add time or repetitions to
the exercises as you wish. Certain exercises may be exceptionally
good for you and you may want to include these exercises every
time you practise. This is perfectly satisfactory but do not neglect
the other exercises of the group. If any of the exercises seem to be
more difficult, perform them cautiously and without strain but do
not neglect them. If you are serious in your practice you should
eventually be able to do every one of the exercises. Let me repeat
that the Yoga movements are not 'calesthentics'. Because of the
manner in which you move and practise the Yoga exercises you
slowly and surely change a great deal of your body. As this occurs
there are often minor discomforts and people sometimes become
discouraged because they are looking for impossible sudden
'miracles'. But if you persevere you will be grateful for your entire
life because of the effect that Yoga will have upon you. For complete details regarding practice, re-read the information presented
earlier in the book.

The number in the parenthesis to the left of each exercise in
the practice chart is the number of the exercise, not the page.
You may have to flip the pages in the beginning but very quickly
you will become familiar with the time and repetition for each
exercise.

The pages which follow the chart present very important information regarding this Practice Plan.

LIFETIME PLAN OF PRACTICE

❶

(4) COMPLETE BREATH

(12) STANDING TWIST

(22) RISHI'S POSTURE

(13) ARM AND LEG STRETCH

ABDOMINAL LIFTS

(23a) STANDING
(23b) ALL FOURS
(8) SITTING

(36) CHEST EXPANSION SEATED

(32) FULL TWIST

(5) COBRA

(15) NECK TWIST

(6-16) LOCUST

(17) BOW

(37) SIT UP; LIE DOWN

(39) HEAD STAND (OR SHOULDER STAND)

(40) ALTERNATE NOSTRIL BREATHING

❷

(4) COMPLETE BREATH

(35) KNEE AND THIGH STRETCH

(9) ALTERNATE LEG PULLS

(11) ROLL TWIST

(21) HIP BEND

(10) SIDE BEND

(30) LEG CLASP

(38) LEG OVER

(19) SHOULDER STAND WITH VARIATIONS

(20) PLOUGH

(1) LEG PULLS

(40) ALTERNATE NOSTRIL BREATHING

❸

(4) COMPLETE BREATH

(25a) FINGER EXERCISE
(25b) ELBOW EXERCISE

(31) POSTURE CLASP

(34) NECK ROLL

(14) LION

(26) EYE EXERCISE

(24) SIMPLE TWIST

(3) CHEST EXPANSION

(33) OVERHEAD SQUAT

(27) SIDE RAISE (LEFT SIDE)

(28) BACK PUSH UP

(27) SIDE RAISE (RIGHT SIDE)

(6-16) LOCUST

(29) ALL FOURS

(40) ALTERNATE NOSTRIL BREATHI

INFORMATION REGARDING THE PLAN OF PRACTICE

Complete Breath — This technique should be practised each day you begin your exercises. It can be done seated without raising your arms or standing as depicted in Exercise 4. (The Complete Breath can also be practised in the course of the day's activities, without the exaggerated movements of raising the shoulders and arms.)

Standing Twist; Rishi's Posture; Arm and Leg Stretch — These three postures are all excellent to impart balance, grace and poise. They should be practised in the order presented. Try always to do the Standing Twist on your toes as indicated in the 4th movement of the exercise (No. 12). Rishi's Posture will give you fine co-ordination and help balance the sides. The Arm and Leg Stretch is not easy and you should not become discouraged if you continue to lose your balance at first. Practise with the upraised arm against the wall and gradually move away. You will have a great feeling of satisfaction and control as you accomplish this posture.

Abdominal Lifts — The 3 positions should be practised in the order indicated. Each position has been devised for a different purpose. Note carefully the position of the hands and trunk in the standing posture (23a). The All Fours position is a fine exercise for new mothers. The Sitting position is simple. The 'inset' illustration 23a depicts how your abdomen should be raised. Note the indentation of the throat area. This is only possible if you have exhaled all of the air from your lungs. Among the three positions you should perform at least 100 lifts. These movements have proved to be excellent for constipation. Consult your doctor about this. Naturally the Abdominal Lifts can be performed each day—even several times a day (always with the stomach empty) if you wish.

Chest Expansion Seated — A simple, non-strenuous variation of the standing Chest Expansion for loosening and flexibility. Excellent for the waistline.

Full Twist — One of the most powerful movements for keeping the spine flexible and young. This posture requires a little study to learn the movements correctly. Notice how the thigh locks the lower spine and the upper spine twists against this lock. If the posture is difficult for you as depicted in the illustrations, you can make it easier by pushing the foot and leg away from the knee in movement 4.

Cobra; Neck Twist; Locust; Bow — These four exercises should be done as a group in the order presented. The Completed Locust (16) comes only with practice, but you'll grow stronger each time you try it. The same is true with the Bow. When you can bring your knees up in the Bow, try the gentle rocking movement to and fro (like a rocking horse) 5 times.

Sit Up; Lie Down — Self-explanatory. An excellent firming and muscle toning exercise.

Head Stand — Another exercise which requires patience and practice but very well worth it. Almost everyone can do some form of the Modified Head Stand if they really try. If your neck is weak or if you have high blood pressure, proceed very cautiously or consult your doctor to receive his opinion. If you feel it is absolutely impossible for you to do the Head Stand, substitute the Shoulder Stand in its place.

Knee and Thigh Stretch — Don't be discouraged if you find your knees and thighs stiff when you try this one. The exercise is designed to help stretch and elongate the muscles, ligaments and tendons of the inside of the thighs. Your legs will feel younger as you continue this stretching technique.

Alternate Leg Pulls — Your best exercise for quick relief of tension throughout the legs. Work to be able to place your clasped hands around the foot.

Roll-Twist — An easy exercise for the waistline.

Hip Bend — An easy movement to firm through the sides and upper arms.

Side Bend—Work to rest one hand on the ankle and bring the other arm over your head.

Leg Clasp—A powerful movement for flexibility of the spine and firming the legs. Once accomplished, you should never lose this.

Leg Over—Move the legs slowly and work to bring the leg high toward the head when resting on the floor. You will quickly feel the firming properties of this movement.

Shoulder Stand—A technique that has so many benefits, it is difficult to name them all. Most interesting is the effect on the thyroid gland. As you continue to practise attempt to bring the trunk into a completely vertical position. Variations with the Shoulder Stand are as follows: After holding the vertical position for as long as is comfortable (several minutes), do a slow split with the legs and slowly move them as far as possible to the sides. Next, keeping the legs apart do a slow twisting movement with the trunk, first to the right, then slowly to the left. Next, return to the frontward position and slowly bring the legs back together. Straighten up once again into the vertical position and slowly lower the legs behind you in to the Plough.

Plough—The Plough follows the Should Stand and presents a powerful stretching and firming movement for the spine, entire back and legs. If your legs will not reach the floor, simply hold them at your extreme position. With practice they will gradually touch the floor.

Leg Pulls—This exercise may follow the Plough. From the lying position slowly sit up without the use of your hands and perform the Leg Pulls.

Finger and Elbow Exercises—Self-explanatory. For purposes of keeping the joints flexible.

Posture Clasp—Excellent for the arms and for relieving tension in the shoulders. If hands will not reach one another use a piece of cloth.

Neck Roll—Perform slowly to keep the neck tension-free. troubled with neck tension perform both the Neck Twist and Ne Roll exercises.

Lion—For best results, don't hesitate to become ferocious a really stick out your tongue. Good muscle tone in the face will he to keep the skin from sagging.

Eye Exercise—Self explanatory. Open the eyes wide as you pe form these movements.

Simple Twist—For a quick and non-strenuous loosening of t spine.

Chest Expansion—A powerful movement for quick relief of tensi throughout the entire body. May be done anytime of the day f revitalisation.

Overhead Squat—A slow and graceful deep-knee bend for balan and firming of the legs. The hands are above the head, not resti on it.

Side Raise; Back Push Up; Side Raise; Locust; All Fours These five exercises form a powerful firming routine and shou be performed in the order presented. You can warm up for the Si Raise by lifting only one leg the first time. Then bring up both leg keeping the knees straight and with the feet touching. Rememb to arch your neck in the Backward Bend. This enables you to pu up further. After doing the Side Raise on the right side, roll ov on the abdomen and perform the Locust. The entire routine of the four movements can be done two to three times. Finish the routi with the All Fours exercise by bringing your hands in beneath yo shoulders at the completion of the Locust and lifting yourself grac fully into the All Fours starting position. With each repetition of t All Fours, bring your hands in further toward your knees so that y are eventually in the position of the 3rd movement.

Alternate Nostril Breathing—One of the most powerful natu tranquillisers for mind, body and emotions ever devised. Ma certain the count is steady and rhythmic. Once learned, this tec nique will become one of your best friends in times of stress. It excellent to finish each day's practice with this breathing exercis

The following tables indicate the exercises and techniques to which you can devote special attention if you are attempting to overcome a particular problem. The exercise number is indicated in the parenthesis. These suggestions are offered strictly from the viewpoint of the Yoga exercises and are not to be used as a substitute for medical treatment. If in doubt regarding the effect of any of the exercises, consult your doctor.

FACE (Muscles strengthened, complexion improved)

Lion (14)
Chest Expansion (3)
Locust (6) (16)
Shoulder Stand (19)
Backward Bend (2)
Eye Exercise (26)
All Fours (29)
Neck Roll (34)
Head Stand (39)

FEET (Ankles, Toes, loosened, strengthened)

Backward Bend (2)
Toe Twist (12)
Lotus Postures (7)
Overhead Squat (33)
All Fours (29)

HEADACHES (Relieved)

Directing the Life-Force (18)
Complete Breath (4)
Shoulder Stand (19)
Chest Expansion (3)
Eye Exercise (26)
Neck Roll (34)
Chest Expansion Seated (36)

LEGS (Thighs, firmed, strengthened, tensions relieved)

Leg Pulls (1)
Alternate Leg Pulls (9)
Plough (20)
Locust (6) (16)
Bow (17)
Backward Bend (2)
Rishi's Posture (22)
Side Raise (27)
Back Push Up (28)
All Fours (29)
Overhead Squat (33)
Knee and Thigh Stretch (35)

LUNGS (Expanded, cleansed)

Complete Breath (4)
Chest Expansion (3)
Directing the Life-Force (18)
Backward Bend (2)
Chest Expansion Seated (36)
Alternate Nostril Breathing (40)

NECK (Strengthened, tension relieved)

Neck Movements (15)
Cobra (5)
Backward Bend (2)
Shoulder Stand (19)
Plough (20)
Back Push Up (28)
Neck Roll (34)

NERVOUS SYSTEM (Nervousness, Insomnia, tension relieved)

Complete Breath (4)
Cobra (5)
Neck Movements (15)
Chest Expansion (3)
Directing the Life-Force (18)
Neck Roll (34)

POSTURE (Corrected, Improved)

Cobra (5)
Chest Expansion (3)
Backward Bend (2)
Bow (17)
Posture Clasp (31)
Chest Expansion Seated (36)

SCALP (Stop Falling Hair, retain lustre, color)

Chest Expansion (3)
Shoulder Stand (19)
Backward Bend (2)
Rishi's Posture (22)
Leg Clasp (30)
Head Stand (39)

SPINE (Stiffness relieved, strengthened)

Chest Expansion (3)
Backward Bend (2)
Cobra (5)
Locust (6) (16)

SPINE (Continued)

Bow (17)
Plough (20)
Rishi's Posture (22)
Leg Clasp (30)
Full Twist (32)
Chest Expansion Seated (3

WEIGHT (In conjunction w proper nutrition)

Reduced in Waist and Hips

Abdominal Movements (8)
Shoulder Stand (19)
Plough (20)
Roll-Twist (11)
Abdominal Lifts (23)
Hip Bend (21)
Full Twist (32)
Chest Expansion Seated (3(
Sit Up; Lie Down (37)
Leg Over (38)

Reduced in Buttocks, Thighs and Leg

Shoulder Stand (19)
Cobra (5)
Locust (6) (16)
Complete Breath (4)
Side Raise (27)
Back Push Up (28)
All Fours (29)
Overhead Squat (33)
Sit Up; Lie Down (37)
Head Stand (39)

This part of the book is written primarily for those people who have become interested in and are practising physical Yoga. It may be unlike anything you have ever read before regarding foods, diet and nutrition in general.

Yoga is a way of life and nutrition is one part of this way. If you have been practising your Yoga exercises with me during our television programmes and have followed the general plan of practice which I have presented, you cannot help but begin to feel the sense of what I refer to as a 'new life'. It is very hard for us to put our finger on exactly what this feeling is. Some of the terms that might be applied are 'exhilaration', 'elation', 'optimism' or perhaps simply 'a general sense of well being'. The reason that this is true is because you are stimulating and awakening a great amount of force and power which has been asleep within you and which you ordinarily do not use. As this force is aroused, you begin to function more energetically, harmoniously and as a better integrated human being. This can be compared to an eight cylinder automobile which has been running on only two cylinders and is gradually given back the power of the cylinders which have not been functioning; the increase in energy and efficiency is pronounced. Now, in order to keep these cylinders operating to their fullest capacity, it is important, in addition to our Yoga exercises, to consider the subject of nutrition and to see how essential a wholesome and nutritious diet can be.

During my nutritional talks on television I have presented a great amount of information pertaining to what you should be getting from the foods you eat. From the Yogic viewpoint I have told you the best manner for the preparation and cooking of many foods and have given you menus and recipes to make eating both interesting and nutritious for you and your family. There have been a great many requests from viewers to put these ideas in written form so that they may be referred to as desired. This is exactly what I have done in this book, and the result is a manual packed with information which has been gained from my experience with thousands of Yoga students. I know you will derive great benefits from this knowledge. It is no exaggeration to state that it would probably take you many years and a great deal of money to discover for yourself the information contained herein. Therefore, keep this manual handy where you can read it often and refer to it when needed. As you begin to absorb this knowledge and change your eating habits in accordance with the principles which have been established for proper nutrition, you should certainly accelerate your progress in the entire practice of Yoga.

Many of our television students have already begun to experience the connection between proper nutrition and what we are attempting to accomplish with our Yoga exercises, and it seems virtually impossible for any person who is seriously concerned with developing the health of body and mind not to realise sooner or later that nutrition must play an important role in this effort.

I have explained both in previous chapters and during our programmes, that from the Yoga viewpoint, all life is sustained by a force which the Yogis have named **prana**. We can translate this Sanskrit word **prana** into English by using the term 'life-force'. We have used this life-force in a number of ways. One of our most important Yoga techniques consists of 'Directing the Life-force' which I explained earlier in the book. All living things must continually receive life-force to sustain themselves. This is true throughout the human, animal and vegetable kingdoms. The more life-force which an organism contains, the higher the quality of life. When the life-force is insufficient or is unbalanced, the quality of life is poor, and physical, mental and emotional disturbances occur. The Yogi thinks of many illnesses and disorders in terms of an insufficient quantity of life-force in the organism. When the amount of life-force begins to fall below that which the body must have, various compensations and adjustments are made by the organism in an attempt to regain the proper balance Your body will make you rest or sleep; it will require that you eat more or less (in accordance with what it is attempting to accomplish); it will make you drink fluids; it will give you the desire for heat or cold, etc. In other words, the intelligence of your body will make you do everything possible to maintain an adequate supply of life-force. If you comply with its needs, the Yogi believes you will succeed in your Yoga practice and that you will grow and develop mentally, emotionally and spiritually. Thus, the Yoga formula is as follows: the more life-force, the more awareness of 'life' and all its implications; the less life-force, the less sense of 'life' and the realisation of its meaning and purpose.

How do we insure an adequate and continued supply of life-force? Do we drink a few cups of coffee, take a 'pep' pill, buy some 'miracle' machine or gadget that gives us what we need? "No," says the Yogi, "these things fool you temporarily into thinking or feeling that something is being accomplished, but the illusion is dispelled sooner or later when you begin to realise that the coffee may be damaging your nervous system, that the 'pep' pill is simply quickening your metabolic activity and that the machine is at the very best only a temporary crutch." The Yogi does not believe that there is life-force in such things. Where then is the life-force? In order to understand these vital energies and their connection with nutrition, it is important to consider briefly the other sources from which we derive our life-force and see what conclusions we may draw.

If you walk into a room which is full of gas fumes you will either open the windows and doors to let in the fresh air or you will leave the room immediately. No one has to tell you that you are breathing impure or 'dangerous' air. You are immediately aware that if you stay and breathe the fumes of the gas your life-force will be quickly depleted and your life will expire. You can tell when you are breathing smog or high carbon dioxide or fumes, and you can also tell the difference in how you feel when your are breathing the fresh, pure air of the seashore of the very finest air of the mountains. Conclusion: **pure air has the most life-force and mountain air is the purest air.**

Nobody has to tell you when it is time to go to sleep. Your body says to you, "Our life-force level is low, you must therefore temporarily cease your activities and pass into the state of sleep so that we may rebuild and raise the level of the life-force." You are tired and you go to sleep. If you sleep the correct number of hours (which differs with each individual) you awaken 'well rested', and you are able to attend efficiently to the things you must do because both your body and mind are alert and sharp. But many people ignore the sleep demands of the body because they think they are doing something more important with that time. Then again, there are those who, although going to bed in time to get a good night's rest, cannot sleep because they have already so depleted their life-force in another aspect of their living (emotionally, mentally) that they lie awake or toss and turn and the results are obvious in both cases: inability to accomplish efficiently what must be done; irritability, fatigue, nervousness. If a person in this situation continues to ignore the body's sleep requirements and thus depletes his life-force more and more he must eventually have a 'breakdown' of one kind or another. Conclusion: **your body will always let you know when it requires sleep to replenish its life-force.**

If you detect that water is polluted or impure you will not drink it because you know it will prove harmful to the organism. The point is that we seem to have a great intuitive knowledge concerning the requirements of the life-force in regard to the elements of air, sleep, water and others which it is not necessary to go into here. But it is when we come to **foods** that we find ourselves in trouble because in the matter of foods we often seem to trust wholly to our taste buds; if foods 'taste good' and fill up the stomach we feel that the primary requirements are satisfied. But the body must derive a great deal of its life-force from foods and if it does not receive what it should it will gradually begin to break down. Of course, this 'breakdown' may take years to materialise and so when we finally find ourselves ill the last thing to which we are inclined to attribute our illness is the years of neglect, abuse and poor nutrition which has finally produced the negative condition. The body has actually fought long and hard to prevent the illness and has tapped every available source to acquire sufficient life-force, but it is finally unable to continue and you have a situation where the engine has simply run out of fuel. Naturally, we would like to **prevent** this breakdown, especially when an individual is still relatively young in years, and the Yogi believes that through the Yoga exercises, proper nutrition and sensible living habits, this can be accomplished. But it must be remembered that there is much more than simply the physical well-being which is involved; there are great philosophical and spiritual implications when one maintains his body as 'the temple of the spirit'.

Since we are already engaged in the process of learning and practising the Yoga exercises, learning proper breathing and how to relax and obtain a restful night's sleep, let us now concentrate on gaining life-force through proper nutrition.

One of the questions which I am most frequently asked is, "What does the Yogi eat?" However, the important thing for us is not **what** the Yogi eats but **why** he eats! "Well," you may say, "he must eat for the same reason anyone does—in order to live." To a certain extent this is, of course, true. But the Yogi feels that it is not enough simply to 'eat to live'. He wants to sustain a **high quality of life** and he is very much aware that foods have a great deal to do with the quality of life. Do you suspect that this is true? When the Yogi selects his foods, what he is really asking himself is, "Do these foods contain life-force?" Sometimes you know if you have eaten a meal that contained life-force foods that truly provided you with nourishment by the way you feel after eating. The Yogi's foods will always leave him feeling 'light' and 'alive'. He **wants** to remain light and energetic, not heavy, dull and lethargic. Therefore, he eats small quantities of high quality, life-force foods. It is the Yogi's belief that, within reason, the less you eat, the healthier you will feel, the more energetic you will be and the longer you will live without complications, providing that your foods are of a high quality. More illnesses than we know are probably caused by indiscriminate and/or continuous over-eating. The fact that you do not immediately drop dead after finishing one of our usual seven course dinners may not mean that you are receiving adequate nourishment from that meal. It is, rather, a testimonial to the tremendous strength of the organism, to how much abuse it can take day after day, year after year and still survive. But there may come a time when the digestive organs can no longer cope with what you have been pouring into yourself at least three times each day and then you may find yourself in serious difficulty. Of course, very few people think to place the blame on years of this type of eating for their physical or emotional distress. A 'virus' or a 'neurosis' seems to be much more handy and sophisticated.

Now, lest these statements be misinterpreted, we must add that illnesses are not necessarily the result of improper nutrition, but we do believe very strongly, along with many of our country's leading nutritionists, that a great deal of illness could be **prevented** through proper nutrition. There has been a tremendous amount of research and experimentation in the field of nutrition and there are a great number of facts to lend substance to the above statements. However, we do not consider it necessary to present any documentation here, primarily because this manual is strictly for students of Yoga who have already begun to experience and understand the nature of life-force and some of its implications through the exercises and techniques we have been practising. This book is not meant to 'convince' anyone of anything. The information is offered to you as a supplement to your Yoga study. If you are in doubt as to how any of the menus or suggestions will affect you, you must always consult your doctor. If you are under the care of a doctor you should certainly consult him before undertaking any of the menus offered in these pages.

As we present our Yoga concept of foods and life-force, you may get the idea that you are going to be asked to restrict yourself, through the use of your will power, to a type of eating which is unpleasant. In other words, there is going to be a kind of 'battle' between what you really **want** to eat and what you **shoul** eat. Nothing could be further from the truth. It is not our in tention to deprive you of the 'fun' of eating, but rather to demon strate that nutritious eating may not only be more delightful tha your current diet, but that the benefits of your entire Yog programme can help to make you a better person, both in bod and mind.

There may be many foods which you might now like t eliminate from your diet—things such as refined sugar products sweets, cakes, stimulants such as coffee and perhaps even smoking This all becomes possible when you apply the principles of sensibl eating. This is true because the body begins to cleanse itself from the influence of the above things; the life-force is stimulated and greater intelligence (which the Yogi refers to as the 'wisdom o the body') begins to operate more actively within you. You ma then begin to lose your taste for such things. I have never told student to 'stop smoking' or 'stop eating sweets' although I know it would be extremely beneficial for him to do so. This is lik saying to someone, "You must relax!"; "I know I must", answer the dismayed person, "but **how?**". I have found out long ago tha it is highly inadvisable for the student to either force or auto suggest himself into giving up a food or a habit to which he is ver attached. Have you ever tried telling a coffee addict to stop drink ing coffee? Your advice may be appreciated but will produce n results. If the coffee addict needs two or three cups to get hi eyes open in the morning and a few coffee breaks during th day to consume another three or four cups, lest he or she ru amuck and do in his fellow workers or the children, then he is no going to give up his coffee. The same is true for the smoker wh becomes panicky and is on the verge of a nervous breakdow when he finds himself out of cigarettes. But I will tell you a stonishing fact. Many of my class students and television viewers have stopped their coffee, cigarettes and many harmful eating habits because, "I simply lost my taste for it!". As the life-force grows more active through our various Yoga techniques, it seems that one automatically cultivates a taste and desire for those foods which he knows intuitively will prove truly nourishing. This is something that can only be **experienced**, not debated or intellectually discussed. The Yogi is not concerned with whether or not you have 'faith' or believe what we are saying or whether you are armed with a great number of technical arguments and theories. If you are attracted to the entire concept of Yoga in general, simply try what we are suggesting along the nutritional lines. The results will speak for themselves.

You have probably heard me remark frequently that "Yoga is a way of life." In this way of life we find that we are inclined to be drawn more and more toward everything which is 'natural' and to become in tune with nature. This idea carries over into our foods and eating habits. For example, it is the theory of the Yogi that most **natural** foods (foods which grow and certain dairy products) are exceptionally rich in life-force. Our objective now is to select foods which are richest in life-force and to prepare them in a manner which will preserve as much of this life-force as is possible. Let us examine the various classifications of foods and determine how this can be accomplished.

Practically all fruits are a source of energy which is derived from their natural sugar content. In addition, they are excellent for cleansing purposes and often contain many vitamins and minerals. It is unfortunate that so many people regard fresh fruits as little more than an accessory to their diets; as a snack between meals or as an occasional dessert. It is the Yogi's belief that fresh fruits, as available, should constitute a major part of one's daily diet. Fruits are, for the most part, easily digested and are a quick source of heat and energy which is very much in keeping with our idea of conservation of energy and placing the least possible burden on the digestive organs. We can classify the various fruits which are available to us at different times of the year as follows:

ACID FRUITS (also known as citrus fruits)—These include oranges, grapefruits, lemons, tangerines, pineapples, pomegranates and such berries as the strawberry, loganberry, cranberry. Many of the acid fruits are sub-tropical fruits since they require that climate for growth. The orange and grapefruit can probably be considered as exceptionally important because of their content of vitamin C. Vitamin C is a vital element which does not store in the body and must therefore be provided daily. It is interesting to note that although we refer to these fruits as 'acid' fruits, they actually have an alkaline effect once consumed. The orange is a fruit which is exceptionally high in fruit sugar. This sugar is ready for immediate assimilation. The grapefruit is excellent for cleansing purposes as is the juice of the lemon and lime. Many students have eaten only two or three grapefruits for breakfast for a week at a time and have found the resultant feeling of lightness and alertness to be most gratifying. You may wish to experiment with this idea not only for cleansing but for reducing purposes. It is important to add that if you are going to give this plan a fair trial you must not combine the acid fruits with the usual foods used at breakfast, i.e., eggs, ham, bacon, toast and coffee. As far as we are concerned in this study, the acid fruits do not combine well with these foods. You cannot expect the citrus fruits to be truly effective for our purposes of cleansing when these other food elements are introduced together with oranges, grapefruits and their juices. The citrus fruits combine well with each other and can be mixed with certain proteins such as nut butters. This is indicated in the menus which appear later.

I would like to offer a suggestion which has proved very valuable for many students. Upon rising in the morning, mix the juice of a half lemon with about 4 ounces of bottled spring water. Wait for several minutes and then perform the ABDOMINAL LIFT exercise, which is illustrated earlier in the book. You may find that this procedure will have an excellent effect on improving elimination. Lemon and lime juice contain alkaline elements and citric acid. These juices should also be used frequently as salad dressings which are indicated in our menus and recipes. I would not advise the use of any sweetening agent (honey, sugar, etc.) with citrus fruits. All citrus fruit juices are excellent and will provide varying amounts of vitamin C. These juices should be freshly squeezed either by you or where you can see it done, since we know that a great deal of value is lost if the juice stands for even a half-hour. If fresh citrus fruits cannot be obtained, frozen juices are our next choice.

SUB-ACID FRUITS—This category includes fruits such as apples, apricots, peaches, cherries, plums, grapes, melons, papaya, mangoes, etc. There are also sub-tropical and tropical fruits such as the banana and avocado that are in this group. When fresh fruits are in season it is often desirable to make these fruits a complete meal. One may eat as many of the sub-acid fruits as he wishes. Such a meal will always leave you feeling light and alert

and these can be supplemented with certain proteins and othe substances so that you will not feel hungry. Many people will ea only fresh fruits, both acid and sub-acid, together with their juice for several days during one of the summer months for purpose of cleansing. This is sometimes referred to as a fruit 'Fast' and wi be explained in more detail later. There is a popular misconcep tion on the part of many people regarding such fruits as banana and avocados. It is thought that the elements which compos these fruits must make one 'fat'. The oils and fats which are con tained in these foods are necessary and highly beneficial an should not add excess weight **if correctly combined wit compatible foods.** People who will eat an avocado salad wit what is already a steak and potato dinner of high calorie conten cannot place the blame on the avocado for adding extra pounds

DRIED FRUITS—The principal fruits in this category are th date, fig and raisin. These are wonderful sources of immediat sugar energy. They can be used very satisfactorily as a substitut for refined sugar products, including sweets, cakes and othe 'snacks' for between meals. Children should be encouraged t eat these rather than sweets and cakes. They make an excellen lunch-box item. Other fruits can also be 'dried', such as th apricot, peach and the plum (which becomes the prune). mixture of dried fruits soaked overnight in water, makes a excellent breakfast dish during winter months. Children usuall enjoy raisins and dates with cereals and often with salads. Fron the Yogic viewpoint, one should not consume the dried fruit which have been preserved with sulphur dioxide. All health foo stores and many markets and grocery stores now carry th natural dried fruits without preservatives. The dried fruits whicl are free from preservatives also seem to have a much mor wholesome and delicious flavour.

In combining the three categories of fruits listed above, the following principle should be remembered: acid and sub-acid fruits may be combined; sub-acid and dried fruits may be combined; acid fruits and dried fruits should **not** be combined. Remember that all fruits can and should be eaten raw without syrups, sweeteners or preservatives. Dried fruits may be soaked overnight to make them softer and more easily digestible for those people who so desire. Cooking is unnecessary for fruits, although apples may occasionally be baked with a small amount of honey. Fruits may be eaten with certain proteins, particularly cheeses and nuts or nut butters (or other high quality proteins which are indicated in this book). It is also feasible to mix certain fruits with raw vegetables for a nourishing salad; i.e., apples and raisins go well with lettuce, cucumbers, carrots and other bland raw vegetables. You will have no trouble devising an interesting variety of delicious combinations.

Most edible vegetables contain important nutritional elements. Vegetables are generally considered by many people as another 'accessory', as something which is stuck on the side of the plate as a kind of 'ornament' to meals. Very few red-blooded "All-American" men would dare to eat an all vegetable meal since they are sure they could not possibly fill their stomachs or have enough nourishment. The ignorance regarding the tremendous nutritious quality of properly prepared vegetables is widespread throughout the United States. I think that this was beautifully summarised in a classic cartoon which appeared in a well known magazine several decades ago. A mother is standing over a small child who is seated at a table with a dish of greens in front of him. The mother says, "It's broccoli, dear," and the child answers, "I say it's spinach and I say to hell with it!" One can hardly blame this child and the succeeding generations of children (and adults) who have cultivated a strong aversion to vegetables. Why? Because they don't taste good. Why? Because their wonderful natural and subtle flavours are often destroyed in the preparation. Vegetables are actually full of flavour and you can detect this flavour the moment the taste buds are purified. That is, if you eat for several days without condiments or sweeteners or if you eat nothing at all for several hours the taste buds will begin to regain their natural sharpness. Then have a salad, or vegetables which are correctly prepared, and you will be astonished at how flavourful vegetables really are! The greatest mistake made in the preparation of vegetables is the over-cooking. Not only is the natural flavour boiled away, but so is the life-force. Then, in order to compensate for the tastelessness of the vegetables, plenty of salt, pepper and other spices are added. Another fact that is not appreciated is the flavour in **raw** vegetables. Many vegetables which would taste delicious in their raw state lose this flavour through cooking because the housewife has simply never thought to serve these vegetables in their natural state. Or she has become so accustomed to boiling her vegetables in a particular manner that she has never tried under-cooking (tenderising) these vegetables so that their flavour and life-force remains within them. Who can estimate how many wonderful vitamins and minerals in vegetables are washed down the kitchen drain each year?

Let us have a classification of the various types of vegetables.

FRUIT BEARING VEGETABLES — tomatoes, summer squashes, peppers, cucumbers, okra. These vegetables are low in calories and contain varying amounts of potassium, sodium, calcium, magnesium, iron, phosphorus, sulphur. Tomatoes (a good source of vitamin C), peppers and cucumbers can be eaten raw. These vegetables can also be highly cleansing in nature.

STARCH VEGETABLES—potatoes of all kinds, artichokes, winter squashes and others not well known in the United Kingdom. The common variety of white potato is made up of water, a small amount of protein, starch and cellulose. The sweet potato also contains cane sugar. The potato and artichoke are difficult to eat raw. They are valuable foods when baked and the starch will be well used by the body. I do not suggest using butter or any dairy product with a potato since it is our belief that a starch combined with a fat is a combination difficult to digest.

GREEN VEGETABLES—lettuce (all varieties), celery, chard, spinach, endive, mustard leaves, parsley, brussels sprouts, and all other green leafy vegetables. These vegetables are the most valuable as far as life-force is concerned. They should be eaten liberally each day, raw in salads with dressings as indicated in the recipes, or very lightly steamed. Never boil or over-cook these valuable leaves. Even when steamed, they must remain crisp. Mustard greens and cauliflower are vegetables which are not usually eaten raw, but try them with a natural dressing. Steaming time for each of the above vegetables varies but it is a simple matter to learn this.

ROOT AND BULB VEGETABLES—carrots, turnips, onions, beets, parsnips, radishes, garlic, rutabagas, asparagus, horse-radish. Again, these vegetables should only be steamed in preparation. Onions, carrots, radishes and asparagus tips can be eaten raw.

All vegetables of the above classifications can be mixed i any combinations. Vegetables may also be combined with pro teins to good advantage. It is desirable at one meal each day t have both a raw, home made salad seasoned with the dressing indicated in the recipes and one or more steamed vegetable There are also vegetable salt products which are excellent fo adding a little flavour. If you steam a vegetable, make certain tha the water is never thrown away. Either serve it as a drink seasone with vegetable salt, as a broth or as stock for a heavier soup This broth can be refrigerated for perhaps one day, but beyon this time it is doubtful whether it retains much of its life-force

Also remember that whenever possible eat the skin c vegetables, as a great amount of life-force lies next to the skir This is true even of the white potato. Naturally the skins of th sweet potato or the winter squash are too tough for most digestiv systems. The vegetables which you are served in the Chines restaurants are excellent. You may be able to purchase these fror certain stores which cater to these restaurants. Such vegetable as the bean sprouts (indeed, sprouts of all types, including mun bean, alfalfa), Chinese lettuce, cabbage, etc., are excellent. An notice that when they are served to you in these restaurants the are always tender and crisp, never boiled and limp. Of course we do not approve of the type of sauces with which many c these vegetables are served because we feel they are highl irritating to the digestive system, but the manner in which the are cooked is correct.

Fresh vegetables, as they are available, are our first choice Frozen vegetables would be our second choice.

Fresh vegetable juices are an excellent source of life-forc and easily assimilated. I am referring now to juices which hav been pressed or extracted with a vegetable juice machine. These juices can be purchased in certain health food stores and markets but it is not easy to find the actual fresh (not more than twenty-four hours old) vegetable juices. A vegetable juice extractor manufactured by a reputable firm is a good investment. Such a machine is available in almost any large appliance store. This machine extracts juice from the vegetable and you dispose of the pulp, as it is useless once the juice is extracted. I have given you the recipes for a number of drinks which you can make if you have an extractor.

We should say a few words here about 'inorganic' and 'organic' fruits and vegetables. These are terms which refer primarily to the type of soil in which the food is grown. To simplify what has become a rather controversial subject, let me simply state that with organically grown food, the grower has prepared his soil to contain elements which will grow the finest possible plant. In addition, great care is usually taken to harvest these crops so as to retain their highest nutritional and flavour values. Also, such foods are usually not sprayed or fumigated with insect killers. You should certainly take advantage of any opportunity to buy organically grown foods. You will notice the difference in the flavour. If you cannot get organically grown foods, do not worry about it. Simply wash or soak your vegetables well and scrub the skins before preparation.

Finally, a word about the type of utensils which we prefer for cooking. We prefer stainless steel and "descoware" pots. Regarding the pressure cooking devices, you must always remember that the life-force in foods is very delicate and must be treated gently and with care. The higher temperatures involved in pressure cooking have a tendency to actually 'shock' or 'stun' and very possibly dissipate this delicate life-force. If you are interested in the technicalities of this subject you should not hesitate to do the necessary research through your library.

It is desirable in our work to consume dairy foods which have the lowest possible fat content. This will be readily appreciated by anyone attempting to reduce excess weight. Non-fat or 'skim' milk is probably the best milk for adults. Milk and dairy products in general are high in calcium and protein but are by no means the only source of these elements nor may they be the best source as many people have been led to believe. However, those adults who enjoy milk should use the skim milk. Children can also drink low-fat milk. It is believed by many nutritionists that milk can be highly mucous forming and we have learned from mothers in our classes and viewers of our television programmes that when they cut down on the number of dairy products and increased foods which are high in vitamin C, their children had a noticable decline in the discomforts of colds. If the child is not prone to colds, or if an adult wishes to gain weight, raw certified milk (milk which has been properly inspected but not homogenized and pasteurized) and goat's milk (which is milk of exceptionally high quality) can be obtained from some dairy companies and are excellent products. Both soybean milk and coconut milk are fine products.

The so called 'sour' milk and sour milk products are rich in lactic acid and contain other agents which aid in digestion and elimination. Clabber milk (sometimes known as 'sour milk'), buttermilk and yogurt are all in the family of sour milk products. Yogurt in its various forms has been used for centuries by peoples of the Balkan countries and has become increasingly popular in the United Kingdom in the past decade as more and more people have realised its value. Some health food stores sell the 'culture' with which it is possible to make one's own yogurt. Homemade yogurt is a most delicious food. However, practically every market and grocery store carry not only the plain (vanilla) yogurt but also strawberry, prune and pineapple flavoured yogurts to make them palatable for almost everyone. Yogurt goes well with all fruits and makes an excellent topping for many dishes. Sour cream, although partially a sour milk product, must be considered as exceptionally high in fat content, hence not a desirable food from the Yogic point of view. Butter and cream cheese are products also high in fat content and must therefore be used sparingly.

Cream is, of course, high in fat content. Pure cream used occasionally with fruits or cereals will not be harmful. Occasionally, ice-cream is a good dessert, especially if you can make your own, using raw sugar or honey, pure cream and natural flavouring in place of refined sugar and artificial flavouring. It is possible to buy this type of high quality ice-cream in certain health food stores in the big cities.

Most cheeses are subjected to processing which makes them undesirable for us. They are high fat, aged and usually highly seasoned with salts and other agents. Low-calorie cottage cheese, farmer cheese, hoop cheese, ricotta cheese and all other natural unsalted, skim or whole-milk cheeses are best. All of these cheeses go well with fruits and vegetables and are fine sources of protein, as well as being reasonably low in fat content.

It is very interesting to note that the word 'protein' is of Greek derivation meaning 'primary' or 'holding first place'. This is an indication of the great importance of proteins as far as our diet is concerned. There is currently great stress being placed on the necessity of having an adequate daily intake of protein, and that is as it should be since proteins are the building materials of which all living tissue is made. You need proteins to **lose** weight as well as to **gain** weight! You need protein for vitality and vigour as well as for the health and beauty of the skin, hair and nails. Protein repairs and rebuilds tissues, muscles, glands, nerves, bones and blood, consequently it is needed in convalescence. The child needs protein to grow and the senior citizen needs protein to replace aging and worn out tissues.

However, from our Yogic viewpoint, it is not enough simply to know that you must have protein. There are different types and qualities of protein and it has been my experience that the person not versed in the study of nutrition or bio-chemistry is unaware of the existence of these different types of protein. The average person has generally been led to believe that if he eats plenty of meat, for example, he will be getting all of the protein that is necessary. This may lead him to eat meat three times per day. But the protein in meats is very filling and this will possibly prevent him from eating other foods that contain desirable proteins.

Protein consists of about 50% carbon, some hydrogen, oxygen, nitrogen, traces of sulphur and occasionally phosphorus and iron. And from these elements nature builds **amino acids**. The quality of a protein is determined by the number of amino acids present. There are currently 23 known amino acids, 8 of which are considered essential. Meats and eggs eaten sparingly as will be suggested in our 'Menus', whole milk and whole milk products, yogurt, cheeses, nuts and nut butters, legumes, avocados, dried olives and garlic, should supply the necessary protein

From the Yogic viewpoint, we prefer to obtain as much of our protein as possible from natural foods, that is, foods other than meat products. We do not wish to set a bonfire in the body with high energy foods and have to feed a huge flame whenever it begins to die; we want a small, steady controlled flame. That is why we want simply the adequate amount of high-quality protein.

Let us look into the major sources of natural protein.

NUTS—Almost all nuts are fine sources of protein, but from the Yogic viewpoint they should be eaten unroasted and unsalted and this is especially true when they are eaten after a meal. Almonds, pecans, cashews, brazils, coconuts, pistachios and walnuts are extremely high in protein and combine well with all fruits. Several ounces of nuts, according to the amount of muscular activity one does, should provide sufficient protein at any one meal. They should be chewed very thoroughly. Nut butters are delicious and also rich in protein. Almond and cashew butters are currently available in health food stores and many markets but these should also be unroasted. One to two tablespoonfuls with fruits or vegetables is adequate protein for a meal. In connection with nuts we should also mention **seeds** which are high in protein. Caraway, mustard, poppy, sunflower, pumpkin and sesame seeds are pleasant and nourishing. They should be unroasted and unsalted and can be sprinkled on many fruit and vegetable dishes. A handful of any of the above seeds will provide high quality protein. Do not be afraid of the fat content in nuts and seeds. The body uses fats to supply heat and energy. However, you should not overeat or consume other processed foods also containing fats and oils along with the nuts.

LEGUMES—In this category we find foods such as peas, dried beans (blackeye, lima, kidney), soy beans, lentils, garbanzas, St. John's bread and dried peas. One good serving of legumes can often provide sufficient protein for a meal. In preparing legumes, it is usually desirable to soak them overnight, then bring the water to a boil and let simmer until edible. Legumes can be used as a substitute for vegetables in stews and soups. The soy bean and its by-products are exceptionally nourishing foods and usually high in protein content. Crushed soy beans will produce soy 'milk' which has been used for centuries by Orientals. It is very high in protein. St. John's bread is a food in which the pod is eaten and the bean discarded. It is wonderful for giving the teeth a good work-out. When St. John's bread is ground, it becomes a fine flavouring powder known as 'carob' powder and will make a type of malt base for nourishing drinks (see 'Drinks'). Outdoor workers should consume more legumes than sedentary workers.

CHEESES The values and types of cheeses have already been explained under 'Dairy Products'.

GRAINS, CEREALS, BREADS, ETC.—Whole grains provide another good source of protein as well as being rich in certain vitamins (especially the B complex) and many minerals. It is essential from the Yogic point of view to eat only **whole grain** cereals (either cooked or dry), **brown** rice and **whole grain** breads. In other words, grains and flours should not be denatured, refined or bleached. Whole grain cereals and breads, made from wheat, rye, barley, oats are now available in practically all markets. The whole grain cereals (cooked or dry) can be served as a breakfast food several times each week with certain fruits and milk or yogurt. Children should be encouraged to eat these breakfast foods and discouraged from consuming the refined dry cereals which some nutritionists have labeled "sugared cardboard". Brown rice can also make an excellent breakfast food and is extremely nourishing, especially in cold weather. There are now many wonderful and delicious whole grain breads made from various types of flour and mixtures of flour. At one time, bread was known as the "staff of life" since it contained so many of the vital elements necessary for good nutrition which came from whole grains. When the refining process was perfected, bread became a handy item for mopping up the gravy, which was about all it was good for. But more recently it has again become possible to buy high quality breads, although a relatively small percentage of the population takes advantage of this. Always read the label on the bread which you buy. Make certain that it contains no preservatives and no white, bleached or refined flour. The process of 'refining' is possibly one of the most destructive concepts that has ever occurred in the field of nutrition. Rolls and pastries made with refined flour and sugar are equally undesirable. Unrefined flour and sugar make delicious, wholesome rolls, cakes, cookies and muffins which are also far more flavourful than the white flour products. These can be bought in health food stores and certain markets and are the only types of pastry which children should be allowed to eat.

Various spaghettis and macaronis which make use of whole grains and vegetables such as whole wheat, spinach and soya are delicious and nourishing products. One must be judicious in selecting the ingredients of the spaghetti sauce to be used; a vegetable mixture using whole tomatoes with herbs (not harsh spices) will make an excellent and healthful sauce.

Our statements regarding these elements can be simple and con-

cise. From the Yogic viewpoint, the less seasoning and spicing the better. Spices are used strictly for catering to the taste buds; they do not bring out the flavour in foods but simply change the natural flavour and will often destroy the life-force value of many foods. Rich, spicy dressings do not enhance the value of salads. Salt does not improve the quality of nuts. Spices produce irritation. The Yogi feels that this irritation leads to agitation and restlessness. As your taste buds become cleansed through proper diet, you will need less and less seasoning for your food, since it will be unnecessary to improve upon the natural flavour. In the recipies of this book, we have suggested the addition of mild spices to certain dishes in order to cater to acquired tastes. These spices should be used moderately and gradually decreased as you find yourself needing them less and less. Certain spices and herbs are less irritating than others. For example, such seasonings as basil and thyme are more mild than mustard or pepper. Ordinary table salt (sodium chloride) should never be used from our viewpoint, but vegetable salts (which you buy in the health food store) are acceptable.

Herbs have been used for centuries by all civilizations throughout the world. The values of many herbs are available to us in the form of delicious herb teas which can be purchased from the health food stores.

Hardly any discussion these days of nutrition would be complete without including the controversial subject of the role of cholesterols in the body and the relationship of saturated fats to them. The role of unsaturated fats in body metabolism has not yet been sharply defined. However, logic seems to indicate (and this follows the Yoga thought) that if there is a choice it may be more desirable to use the unsaturated oils. Vegetable oils such as safflower oil, pure olive oil, sesame seed oil and others are available in the health food stores and many markets, and should be used rather than the saturated fats which are common in animal products. These oils may be used in salad dressing and in cooking.

The consumption of sweets, cakes, soft drinks and other products which contain the usual refined white sugar should be kept to an absolute minimum. From our Yogic viewpoint, here are the sweetening agents which are best: molasses (rich in iron), honey (used moderately as it is a very concentrated sweet and make sure that the label on the bottle reads 'natural and un- cooked'), raw sugar (which may not look lily white because it has not been subjected to 'refining'), brown sugar (which is just a shade better than refined white sugar). Cane sugar is a wonderful source of sugar providing it is eaten in its natural form, i.e., the cane stalk itself. The low calorie sugar 'substitutes' such as saccharin and its by products are not satisfactory from our view- point because they are coal tar products. There are many argu- ments pro and con regarding the relative merits and demerits of coal tar. However, there exists so much literature written by nutritionists, as well as by members of the medical profession, for more than fifty years claiming that saccharin can be harmful to the organism, that I see no need to take the chance with its consumption if you have not only natural but nutritious sweet- eners through the substances mentioned above, as well as sugar in its purest form, that of fresh fruit.

The Yogi feels that beverages which are artificial stimulants should be consumed most moderately. We have already spoken about coffee in this connection. Caffeine from coffee and the bromine from tea are stimulants which have an effect upon the nervous system that produce the illusion of energy. Therefore, when your body feels the need for more energy you are going to drink another cup of coffee or tea and receive more temporary stimulation, etc. Soon you are drinking four to eight cups or more each day (in which habit you are liberally aided socially and with convenient dispensers everywhere; the 'tea break' is now a national institution). Drinking of this much coffee or tea must eventually have a telling effect on your nervous system. Many people realise that coffee is not good for them, but they don't know how to stop. In other words, they are 'addicted'. The same is true with tea and cola drinkers. We do not ask you to 'stop' any of these drinking habits abruptly. This would have an irritat- ing effect both physically and psychologically. However, it is a good plan to taper off gradually by substituting the drinks listed below for coffee, tea, etc. It has been our experience that through the serious practice of the Yoga exercises and breathing tech- niques, plus proper nutrition, you will experience a decreasing desire for these artificial stimulants.

The beverages which are healthy and delicious and should be used more and more in place of the stimulants are: fruit and vegetable juices, health teas, natural vegetable broths, bouillons, cereal beverages which are low in caffeine and are known as 'coffee substitutes' and the 'Drinks' listed for you in this book.

Regarding alcohol, if you are accustomed to a cocktail several times a week you need not feel that you must discontinue this. Probably the least harmful of all alcoholic beverages is wine, especially white or light red wine. Alcohol has two basic effects: it makes one feel relaxed (relieves tensions) and/or exhilarated.

But most drinkers are aware that both of these sensations are quite illusionary since when either or both of these feelings wear off, the body is left feeling heavy and inert and the mind usually dulled and depressed. The dependence upon alcohol for the sense of relaxation and exhilaration is, from the Yogic viewpoint, unwise and unnecessary. The natural elation, optimism and exuberance of the organism with an abundance of life-force cannot be duplicated by any intoxicant or drug. Again, as you follow your Yoga routine you will almost certainly notice that the desire for all artificial stimulants, including alcohol, automatically declines. You must experience this wonderful, natural exuberance and joy to truly understand what is involved.

As a final word regarding beverages, we should state that no drink (or food for that matter) should ever be consumed at extreme temperatures: ice cold or boiling hot.

The subject of meat, fish and poultry is a delicate one. It is extremely difficult in our society to minimise the eating of animal flesh and by-products even if one truly wishes to do so. Meat and meat products are so much a part of all meals, everywhere, that in order to minimise meat eating you have to be extremely determined and impervious to the scoffing of friends and relatives who will tell you that you are a food 'faddist' or simply an out and out 'crackpot'. But let us state the case for minimising the consumption of meat from the Yogic viewpoint and then you can decide how far you may wish to follow along these lines.

The fact is that meat inhibits the activation of the life-force and the resulting elevation of mind and spirit. After a big meat dinner you know that you must rest for a considerable period of time before you can again function normally. Your body is more or less immobile and your mind is dulled. That is why meats should be eaten sparingly. 'Sparingly' can mean dropping from three times per day to once per day or from every day to several times per week.

The best meats are organ meats such as liver, kidneys, brains. These should be broiled and served rare. Other meats should also be eaten as lean and rare as possible. Herbs can be used to season to taste. Never fry or overcook your meats.

For many people, poultry (chicken especially), and fish are the most easily digestible of the animal products. Fish and poultry should be broiled or baked, never fried and no harsh condiments used in preparation. Lemon should be used liberally with all fish since it helps to counteract the acidity.

Smoked and pickled meats and fish are undesirable from our point of view because of the process involved in 'smoking' and 'pickling'. Although there are various amounts of protein in all meat products, practically regardless of the form in which they reach your table, the canned, smoked and pickled meat products should definitely be consumed most sparingly.

There is a very interesting experiment which many Yoga students have found most revealing. You may wish to try it.

As soon as is practical and convenient, set aside a period of thirty days during which you will eat no meat, fish, poultry, eggs or their by-products. You should temporarily substitute other proteins as suggested in the discussion on 'Proteins'. At the end of this thirty day period you have yourself a good meat dinner with ll of the usual trimmings. The intense 'let down' and heaviness that occurs physically and mentally after this meal is so revealing that it has often caused a Yoga student to greatly minimise his consumption of meat. This is a very worthwhile experiment and you should try it as soon as possible. One such experiment is worth a great deal of argument, debate and speculation.

Now it is necessary to state again that I am not saying you will not have great success with your Yoga practice if you eat meat. But Yogis believe that you will experience even greater benefits than you could have thought possible by minimising as much as is practical your consumption of meat and meat products. If you are not certain whether to attempt the thirty day experiment desribed above, you should consult your doctor.

Eggs are acid forming since they contain an excess of nitrogen, fat and phosphoric acid. The yoke is richer in iron than the white and from our point of view, is consequently to be preferred if one enjoys eggs. I consider it tragic that the egg (and some form of preserved or smoked meat) seems to be the national breakfast, since eggs become especially acid forming and possibly constipating when fried or scrambled and eaten with fried potatoes, white toast, butter and the entire horrendous combination washed down with coffee, often containing cream and sugar. The best method for the preparation of eggs is the poached or very soft boiled egg. Eggs should always be combined with some alkaline elements contained in vegetables or fruits. The yolk of the hard boiled egg is also acceptable, especially in a green salad. If one cuts down on the amount of meat he eats, he can increase the consumption of eggs.

This subject is a highly technical one and there is much confusion on the part of the public regarding the merits and requirements of vitamins and minerals. The confusion is added to by the advertising literature of the various vitamin and drug manufacturers. The average lay individual, not technically versed in this field, hardly knows what to believe regarding the claims made for various products. He does not understand the value of the formula of the food supplement he may be buying, and often ends up looking simply for a vitamin 'bargain'.

Vitamins and minerals are constituents of food the same as are carbohydrates, fats, proteins, etc. **The interaction and relationship** of vitamins and minerals is extremely complex and new discoveries and developments are periodical.

As you know, vitamins have been lettered and numbered for identification. It is known that certain vitamins and minerals have essential properties, and the need for a number of these properties has been definitely established. Your best source of vitamins and minerals is a wholesome diet, such as that suggested in this book. Different foods contain varying amounts of vitamins and minerals; some have relatively high quantities of one or more elements, others relatively high quantities of other elements. That is why it is necessary to have a well-rounded, nutritious diet.

The vitamins as they are currently classified are: A, the B family which consists of B-1 (thiamin chloride), B-2 (riboflavin), B-6 (pyridoxine), niacin, pantothenic acid, paraminobenzoic acid, folic acid, inositol, biotin, choline, B-12, and C, D, E and K.

Those minerals, for which a definite need has been established, are calcium, phosphorus, iron, iodine. There are many other minerals, some of which have been termed 'trace' minerals and include potassium, manganese, sodium, magnesium, cobalt, copper, zinc, bromine, mercury, silver, aluminium, chlorine, and others. The importance and requirements of these minerals are under investigation. The vitamin-mineral study is complicated by the fact that some vitamins work in conjunction with other vitamins and/or minerals. For example, vitamin D is necessary for the proper utilisation of calcium; vitamin C is necessary for the utilisation of certain essential amino acids from proteins; phosphorus aids, calcium, etc. Therefore it is possible that people who have increased their intake of one or another vitamin or mineral through certain foods or food supplements may be lacking other vital elements needed to correctly assimilate and use the vitamins and minerals in question.

If you are eating a complete, well rounded, nutritious diet continually, you do not have to be concerned about your vitamins and minerals. Nature, in her infinite wisdom, has supplied all the necessary elements in our natural foods. It is this type of natural food diet which I have attempted to indicate in this book. If you feel that your diet (and that of your family) does not fulfil all of the requirements of proper nutrition, then food supplements (containing the established requirements of all necessary vitamins and minerals) may be in order.

There is a unique approach in Yoga to the ever growing problem of weight control. Overweight has become practically a national tragedy. I am sure you do not have to be presented with the reasons for the absolute necessity of controlling your weight; the implications regarding your appearance, feeling and health are obvious. Nobody wants to be overweight. If you doubt the sincere desire of millions of people to control their weight, look into the statistics regarding the annual sale of gadgets, exercise machines, steam cabinets, enrolments in gyms and beauty salons, books on diet, appetite deterrents and wafers and drinks as substitutes for food. The figures are staggering.

As far as we are concerned in Yoga, each person who is overweight has a special problem. It is not adequate to state that "overweight is caused by overeating and insufficient exercise". This is not only an over-simplification but in many cases misleading. What constitutes 'over eating'? Is it the same for all people? How many people do you know who can eat as many calories as they want and gain hardly a pound? How many people conversely can consume a very small number of calories and still add excess weight? Is the popular belief in calorie counting the answer to weight control? How many people work out in the gyms three times a week, do all the gardening and housework at home, run around frantically keeping their home or office in order and still continue to gain weight? Isn't it true that you continually encounter people who should move the weight on top to the bottom, or the weight on bottom to the top, or the pounds on one side to the other side, etc.?

Here is a statement which may surprise you, but which is very much in keeping with the concept of Yoga: the wisdom and intelligence of your body are much greater than the magazine 'miracle' diets and the calorie counting charts. Our objective in Yoga is to stimulate and awaken this innate intelligence (life-force) so that it can do for us all the things we would like to have done. It is not only unnatural but often harmful and dangerous from the Yogic point of view to attempt to reduce excess weight through the burning produced by 'hi-protein', the steaming bath,

he 'miracle' twenty-one day diet, the substitution of powders
nd wafers for the nourishment of food, the push and pull
adgets and quick, forceful, strenuous calesthentics. What is more,
xcess weight taken off in this manner will return in almost every
ase the moment the programme is discontinued. Why? Because
he procedures mentioned above are unnatural, i.e., they do not
ssist nature's plan; they oppose it!

**Again, let me state that your problem of weight con-
rol is probably completely different than that of your
eighbour's. His eating habits may vary considerably from
ours and we are largely the result of our eating habits.
o do not look to him or her for a solution. Look to your-
elf!** In other words, get back in tune with yourself. How is this
ccomplished? In two ways: (1) through our Yoga techniques;
2) by beginning to observe and understand the reaction which
articular foods and combinations of foods have upon **you**. There
re no two fingerprints among the entire world's population
hich are alike (some 25,000,000,000 fingerprints). How much
ess can two human organisms, considering their incredible com-
lexity, be alike? Therefore, rather than attempt to establish
ard and fast rules regarding the counting of calories, the intake
f protein, etc., let us learn certain **principles** of eating and
utrition which seem to conform to nature's plan and then
xperiment with these principles and their reaction upon our
ndividual organisms. In this way, each of us should be able to
etermine for himself his own path. The most encouraging part
f this idea is that if you will make a sincere effort to find out
hat is best for **you**, your organism will aid you in every possible
ay. You do not have to fight your body; you simply have to
armonise with it and listen to what it is asking of you. Is this
ot the most intelligent method of all?

How do we go about finding out what are the requirements
of our organism? What does it want of us? We must first undertake certain fundamentals which, following along the Yogic lines
of living, I will simply call 'natural' principles of eating. The most
basic of all of these principles is to revert as much as you possibly
can to the eating of natural foods, i.e., foods which are eaten in
a form which is as close to their natural state as digestion permits.
These foods, their combinations and preparation, are being outlined for you in this book. It is the premise of this work that as
you follow a wholesome, natural food programme you should be
able to regain and maintain your correct weight.

Now remember we are talking about **your** correct weight,
not the charts on the scales or those listed in the Sunday supplements. Your correct weight must be based upon your skeleton
and bone structure and certain other factors. If you are large
boned your weight and measurements must be different than
those of one who is small boned. If a large boned woman attempts
to model her measurements after the mannequins of the fashion
magazines she will not only be disappointed but this can actually
prove harmful. What is more, it is unnecessary for a person to
decide that he or she will defy their natural structure and take
on the measurements of a muscle man or a fashion model. If you
will define the natural beauty of your own structure, you will
be astonished at how beautiful you really are. Regardless of your
structure, if your weight is correctly proportioned, your muscles
and skin taut and firm, your posture and carriage erect and you
are 'thinking gracefully' by moving with poise and balance, you
will never appear overweight or underweight. You will reveal
yourself as beautiful, confident, vital and in harmony with nature.
This will be especially true when you radiate the internal health

and optimism which can result from the natural food programme such as we are attempting to outline in these pages.

Another important word to those who have a weight problem: Yoga is not a 'crash' programme and is not meant to produce overnight miracles. It has probably taken you many years to acquire a weight problem, especially excess weight, and you must be sensible and allow nature to progress methodically with her gradual but certain plan. Nature cannot be fooled, tricked or compromised. I feel quite certain that most of my viewers and students have come to learn of the folly of 'spot' reducing machines, 'miracle' diets and the various 'crash' programmes.

Finally, any **serious** weight problem should always be dealt with by your doctor and you should always consult him before you undertake any special food programme. If you are not certain as to what your correct weight should be according to your structure, again your doctor should be consulted. But for the average problem of weight control it is our contention that the practice of your Yoga exercises coupled with a sensible food programme is the very best natural procedure you can undertake. It is also important to point out that many of the Yoga relaxing exercises, particularly the breathing and stretching techniques, should pacify and diminish the unnatural desire of the 'compulsive eater'. This desire is often due to nervous disturbances and if the nervousness can be alleviated, the desire may disappear. Underweight people often find that when they are able to relax, their assimilation is much improved. So take heart and give your Yoga exercise and food programme a fair trial of several months. If it doesn't work, you can always return to your old habits. By applying the suggestions in this book you have nothing to lose (except the excess inches and pounds!).

I am including information regarding 'fasting' here because of many letters which I have received from viewers expressing an interest in this subject. To many, the idea of 'fasting' will seem strange and possibly foreign. However, it is a technique of such great age and has been used throughout the centuries to achieve so many physical and spiritual objectives that it is certainly worth one's serious consideration. We must discuss two aspects of fasting: the physical and the spiritual. While for the Yogi it is virtually impossible to separate these two, for purposes of our discussion here, we can make a distinction.

Fasting has been man's most instinctive method of coping with an illness and is used by all animals. When an animal is sick you cannot force him to eat to 'keep up his strength'. He knows instinctively that his recuperative powers are impaired through eating. He will find a quiet place and lie down and not take nourishment until he is well again. Does this not serve as a procedure worthy of note for us? **Fasting is not starving.** When you fast, you voluntarily give up the eating of food for a certain length of time for a particular objective. From the physical standpoint, the fast is undertaken by the Yogi as part of a regeneration programme. It is the belief of the Yogi (as well as numerous groups of health-minded people throughout the world) that when the digestive organs are allowed to rest by virtue of having no food introduced into them, a cleansing process is initiated. This process will continue as long as the fast is prolonged. It is when this process has been completed (the completion being designated by certain indications) that the fast is theoretically terminated. At this point, unless food is again introduced into the organism, the body will start to feed upon itself. This marks the end of fasting and the beginning of starvation. But you may be surprised to know that a long period of time could elapse before this point of starvation is reached. In other words, most people could easily go without food (if they were psychologically prepared so that a false fear of starvation would not be a cause fo disturbance) for many days. This is because the amount of food substances present in the organism at any given time is very great. There are thousands of people throughout America and Europe who each year undertake a prolonged period of fasting (known as a 'complete' fast) for purely cleansing purposes. There are many fascinating stages of the fast, things which occur as the fast proceeds. For example, hunger does not usually increase, it diminishes!

But this is an entire subject in itself and quite a technical one. There are many excellent books written on all aspects of the fast which one can read if interested in the 'complete' fast procedure.

The complete fast as briefly outlined above is, of course, not practical for the average working man and woman. One generally needs long periods of rest during the complete fast. What is practical is the 'partial' fast. This may take two forms. First, you could select a day during which you can rest and relax and eat nothing at all for that day; simply drink water whenever thirsty. You may notice certain negative symptoms such as a temporary headache and some irritability or nervousness. If you busy yourself with certain pleasant activities which you enjoy, these discomforts and that of hunger will be minimised. The next day you would resume eating. If you fasted in this manner once a week the Yogi feels you will be doing your organism a great favour. Try it a few times and see. If you find that the procedure is of value to you then after several weeks of fasting one day you can attempt a two day fast. The fast is always followed by light, natural,

nourishing foods on the following day as suggested in our 'Special' menus. Through this type of 'partial' fasting (and of course, the exercises) you will be undertaking a major part of the Yoga 'regeneration' programme. During the fasting period you drink only water when thirsty. Naturally, it is psychologically important during these days to have as little contact with food as possible. It is helpful to read inspirational literature, mediate and otherwise relax and revitalise the mind. It is not suggested that the fast ever exceed two days without the supervision of an authority.

The second form of the partial fast is the elimination of one or more meals (preferably breakfast) during one or two days, or the drinking of only liquids for several days. Of the three meals eaten daily, breakfast would be the most practical meal to eliminate. In this event you would drink a glass of fresh fruit juice in the morning and eat no solid food until noon. You could go for one or more days drinking only fresh fruit and/or vegetable juices, four or five times each day and varying them as desired. This is a more intense programme of cleansing. You must experiment and see how such a programme would affect you. Some people find themselves feeling light, alert and full of pep and energy. They are able to go two or three days with only the fresh juices. They feel wonderful. Others find themselves quite uncomfortable. The latter must be more cautious in their methods, beginning by fasting for only one meal and gradually extending the length of the fast. Then there is the type of partial fast in which a person can undertake a cleansing programme by eating, let us say, only fresh fruits for one or two days. This would be known as a 'fruit' fast and is best when fresh fruits are in season and plentiful. Water-melons, grapes, peaches and papaya make excellent fruit fasts. If you experiment intelligently you will very quickly be able to work out a programme which is of value to **you**. Again, it is by no means necessary to undertake the fasting techniques in order to succeed with your Yoga programme, but it is a method that has often produced such astonishing results that it must be included in any discussion of Yogic nutrition.

You are undoubtedly aware that in every religious scripture throughout the world there are allusions to 'fasting'. Have you ever wondered about this? I find that many people think that fasting, in its spiritual context, is some sort of denial, discipline or punishment. This is not the case and especially not so from the Yogic viewpoint. During the fast, there is a sensation of elation and spirituality that is difficult to explain and really must be experienced to be understood. But as one ceases to eat, the physical aspect of his existence temporarily becomes less of a reality and he then becomes very aware of the spiritual or (life-force) aspect of his being. This is a most exhilarating, inspiring and joyous experience. Jesus fasted for forty days and nights in the desert. He stated that "Such things come only by prayer and **fasting**." Mahatma Ghandi used the fast as his most powerful force in liberating India from British rule. All of the great saints throughout history in every country of the world have used the fast to gain inspiration and spiritual insight. Think about this and then learn about the force and power of the fast by trying it. From the Yogic viewpoint, all earnest prayer and meditation should always be preceded by a period of fasting.

In the following pages we offer you two types of menus for one full week. Those menus listed under the 'Regular' heading are suitable for the entire family. They make use of the ideas we have been discussing in these pages without being extreme. They should prove to be a new adventure in eating, interesting and satisfying. The 'Regular' menus include the wholesome preparation of many natural foods as well as meat and fish (suggested in moderate amounts). The idea of the 'Regular' menus is that not only will there be no complaining about the lack of foods to which members of the family are accustomed, but there are many new and delicious elements added. The 'Special' menus can be followed by those readers who wish to pursue a diet which is more extreme, i.e., more in keeping with the 'natural' concept of eating. The 'Special' menus should also be undertaken by people who want to control weight and these should definitely be used in conjunction with the partial fast. **We must emphasise that these menus are meant to serve as examples of the type of foods and their combinations and preparations. Many additions and substitutions can be made according to your own ingenuity and inclinations.** You will quickly learn about these as you go along. The basic idea at all times is for you to note continually the reactions which various foods and their combinations have upon **you**. In this way you can modify the suggested menus as necessary.

Most of the ingredients suggested in these menus and the recipes which follow can be obtained from your usual shopping sources. Of course, in light of this discussion you may want to look for markets which could offer you a greater selection of really fresh fruits and vegetables, perhaps organically grown foods, more whole grain breads, natural sweets, herbs and condiments, etc. If you have access to a health food store you should become familiar with the items which are carried in these stores. Whole grain breads, cakes, muffins, dried fruits, herb teas, wholesome sweets, natural oils, fresh fruit and vegetable juices, raw nuts, and see how such a programme would affect you. Some people find natural dressings and even natural cosmetics are products which you will want to try.

In the 'Children's Menus' you will find indications of the type of foods which should be fed to children. When you begin to change the diet of your children they may put up a howl, since they have become accustomed early in life to satisfying their taste buds. They must be taken in hand intelligently and fed (at least at home) foods which will provide them with the real elements of nourishment. Do not stop their former diet abruptly, but make a gradual transition from the devitalised foods to more wholesome foods as suggested in the diet. In this manner the child does not feel he is being deprived of anything.

If you undertake the type of diet as suggested in the following menus, you must give the programme a fair trial of at least several months before you attempt to evaluate its benefits. The organism requires time to adjust to the new diet and to reap its benefits. So do not attempt to make any 'snap' judgments after a few days or weeks, although it has been our experience that most students have begun to experience a general feeling of lightness and well being within approximately one month.

Here are a number of important points pertinent to this discussion:

1. All of the information in this book is to be applied by you with respect to your individual needs and desires. The entire concept of Yogic nutrition is to stimulate, awaken, store and use what we have called 'life-force', and this life-force is to be used not only to rebuild and repair the substances of the body and mind, but also to prevent and resist degenerative forces. It is never too late or too early to undertake the Yogic nutrition programme. The programme is profoundly simple since it seeks only to have man revert, as much as possible, to a 'natural' diet and to prepare and eat foods which would seem to conform to nature's plan.

2. If you have been a heavy meat, starch and sugar eater, or if you are very much overweight, you must adopt the Yogic programme gradually. You can 'taper off' heavy, processed, devitalized foods and the artificial stimulants by using them more sparingly in your diet and eventually eliminating them entirely. The 'Regular' menus provide the best programme for this.

3. **If you are under the care of a doctor, consult him before undertaking any part of the Yogic programme.**

4. Remember that the Yogic nutrition programme works hand in hand with the Yoga physical and mental exercises. For greatest benefits you must undertake the practice of both aspects.

5. Attempt to become in tune with nature in all of your activities. Learn about your physical, emotional and mental 'cycles'; your 'ups' and 'downs' and what cause them. Observe

carefully the physical and emotional reactions which all of nature's elements have upon you, not only in foods as suggested in this discussion, but learn what your requirements are with regard to sleep, exercise, water and sun. Remember you are an individual, different from all other individuals, and you must learn, in the words of the philosopher, to "Know Thyself". Feel and trust the intelligence of your body. If you are not hungry, do not eat, even though the clock says it is dinner time. If you require nine hours of sleep, do not settle for seven. If you find that certain foods and combinations of these foods do not agree with you, do not eat them.

6. Never become a fanatic, a bore or anti-social with your Yogic nutrition programme. It is best to be very quiet and inoffensive about your activities along these lines. If you ever refuse to eat any foods when you are out to dinner or at a social function, do so with a graceful excuse and do not make an issue of your refusal. Never tell another person that the foods which he or she is eating are harmful. You will become very unpopular. You will be branded as a 'food faddist', a 'health nut', etc. We do not wish to 'convince' or force our ideas upon anyone who is not interested or sympathetic with this concept since by so doing we will cause much more harm than benefit. Wait to dispense the information which you have learned in this book and the valuable knowledge which you will gain through your own experiments until you are **asked** why you are looking so radiant and full of vitality. People are certain to notice the change in you because your vibrations will be automatically raised as you gain increased life-force through your Yogic programme of nutrition and Yoga exercises. Everyone around you will feel this increased life-force radiating from you and will undoubtedly begin to question you about it. A comment such as, "You're looking wonderful. What have you been doing?" will be frequent. If you wish, you may mention one or two points about the programme. If you find any scoffing or rejection, simply drop the entire subject. However, if a person appears to be sincerely interested and wants to know more, you may take them into your confidence. But always wait until you are asked. Never volunteer information. When you undertake this programme at home there may be some problems regarding the types of food which you want to eat and those which your family demands. You must simply do the best you can under the circumstances. Always compromise intelligently. Never antagonize.

If you undertake the Yogic menus moderately, gradually substituting the wholesome, nutritious foods for the usual ones, your family may hardly notice the change until they are suddenly aware that they are feeling and looking more 'alive'. You may have to prepare one type of menu for your family and another for yourself, but persevere regardless of the obstacles for at least several months. You cannot afford to disregard the benefits that will be yours. If you ever feel a strong desire for a steak dinner, a hot fudge sundae, candy, hot cakes, spicy foods, etc. go ahead and indulge yourself and do not feel guilty. When you feel satisfied, return to your natural food programme. In this way, you will keep your morale high and will never feel that you are being deprived of something which you crave. When you know you are allowed to eat anything which you really desire, you will be surprised at how often you lose your craving for these foods.

If friends and members of your family poke fun at you for your nutrition programme or your Yoga exercises, it may be because they are secretly envious of your ability to undertake a real self-improvement programme and to display a discipline which they probably lack. Never become irritated with anyone's jibes. If they want to laugh, take it in stride and laugh along with them. Rest assured that you are certain to have the last laugh.

BREAKFAST	LUNCH	DINNER
MONDAY **REGULAR** Dish of steamed brown rice with certified raw milk and honey, raisins. Coffee, herb tea, coffee substitute or Health Drink. **SPECIAL** 1 large grapefruit ½ cup nut butter or whole nuts (unroasted, unsalted) Dish of berries in season. Beverage or Health Drink.	**REGULAR** Carrot juice drink. Avocado and grapefruit salad with ricotta cheese or farmer cheese or cottage cheese; yogurt dressing. Bran muffin. Beverage. **SPECIAL** Vegetable juice combination drink. Salad: romaine lettuce, ½ cucumber, 1 tomato, 2 radishes, 1 stalk celery; french dressing. Rye toast. Cup yogurt with raisins. Beverage.	**REGULAR** Vegetable juice. Lentil loaf. Celery and carrot sticks. Steamed green beans. Applesauce cake. Beverage. **SPECIAL** Tomato juice. Sautéed brains. Green salad; oil and lemon dressing. Cottage cheese dessert. Beverage.
TUESDAY **REGULAR** Cream of rye cereal. Dish of dried prunes soaked overnight; nut butter mixed with juice of prunes. Beverage (as above) **SPECIAL** Dish of sliced peaches, fresh figs, bananas. Cup of cottage cheese topped with raisins, yogurt. Beverage (as above)	**REGULAR** Celery stuffed with cottage cheese and chives. Dish steamed string beans, summer squash, peas, mushrooms; tomato sauce. Wheat toast. Beverage **SPECIAL** Tomato juice. Salad: 1 apple, 2 stalks celery; ½ cup raisins, ½ green pepper; 1 cup cottage cheese; lemon-honey dressing. Dish stewed fruit (dried apricots, prunes, figs soaked in water overnight); wheat germ, yogurt topping. Beverage.	**REGULAR** Broiled liver. Steamed beets with tops. Half head lettuce; yogurt dressing. Banana cake. Beverage. **SPECIAL** Carrot juice. Whole wheat spaghetti. Salad: escarole and lettuce; oil and lemon dressing. Yogurt sherbet. Beverage.

BREAKFAST	LUNCH	DINNER
WEDNESDAY **REGULAR** Dish of sliced oranges. 2 boiled eggs. 1 slice whole wheat health toast; raw butter or health jam. Beverage **SPECIAL** Bunch of grapes in season. Dish of apples, pears and bananas with wheat germ and yogurt topping. Carob milk drink.	**REGULAR** Vegetable Juice drink. Baked vegetable dish: zucchini squash, peas, tomatoes, onion, mushrooms. Banana bread. Beverage. **SPECIAL** Potassium drink. Chives omelet. Rye Toast. Beverage.	**REGULAR** Fresh fruit salad. Broiled fresh fish. Steamed spinach. Apple nut sauce. Beverage. **SPECIAL** Vegetable juice. Broiled liver. Cucumber salad; french dressing. Fresh fruit; yogurt topping. Beverage.
THURSDAY **REGULAR** Whole grain cereal with nut milk, raisins and yogurt topping. Beverage **SPECIAL** Baked apple with honey and wheat germ. Cashew milk (1 cup water; ¼ cup cashews; 2 pitted dates in blender) Oatmeal cookies.	**REGULAR** Bowl vegetable soup. Wheat toast; raw butter. Dish apple sauce with wheat germ, honey, raisins and yogurt or sour cream topping. Beverage. **SPECIAL** Salad: cheddar cheese, sliced figs, apples, grapes, celery on romaine lettuce; chopped almonds. Apple sauce muffin. Beverage.	**REGULAR** Soy bean loaf. Steamed green vegetable. Stuffed celery with cream cheese and chives. Custard pudding. Beverage. **SPECIAL** Pea soup. Apple nut celery salad. Banana bread. Beverage.

BREAKFAST	LUNCH	DINNER

FRIDAY

REGULAR

Orange or grapefruit sections.
2 poached eggs on health bread
(toasted); raw butter or health jam.
Glass raw milk or non-fat milk
(or other beverage

SPECIAL

Dish of sliced oranges, grapefruit,
pineapple and berries in season
with yogurt topping.
Cup of almond or cashew
nuts (unroasted, unsalted)
Fruit milk.

REGULAR

Prunes, raisins, figs, apples, grapes;
cottage cheese; yogurt and
wheat germ topping.
Bran muffin; health jam.
Beverage.

SPECIAL

Salad: escarole and lettuce;
oil and lemon dressing.
Soya wheat bread.
Beverage.

REGULAR

Vegetable juice.
Chicken livers on brown rice.
Green salad; cheddar cheese
dressing.
Honey ice cream; carob cookies.
Beverage.

SPECIAL

Carrot juice.
Stuffed peppers.
Vegetable salad; french dressing.
Baked apple.
Beverage.

SATURDAY

REGULAR

Dish whole grain cereal with wheat
germ, raw milk, bananas.
Bran muffin; health jam.
Beverage.

SPECIAL

Dish of prunes (soaked overnight)
with yogurt topping.
Dish non-fat cottage cheese.
Beverage.

REGULAR

Spanish rice dish.
Green salad; lemon-honey dressing.
Carrot juice or other beverage.
Yogurt sherbet.

SPECIAL

Orange or grapefruit juice.
Dish berries, sliced oranges,
grapefruit; ½ cup almonds or
cashews or 2 tablespoons nut butter
(almond or cashew butter).
Beverage.

REGULAR

Tomato juice.
Steamed fish and chinese
vegetables.
Baked cauliflower; cheese sauce.
Fruit compote; yogurt topping.
Beverage.

SPECIAL

Avocado salad; yogurt dressing.
Stuffed eggplant.
Strawberries with wheat germ.
Beverage.

BREAKFAST	LUNCH	DINNER

SUNDAY

BREAKFAST

REGULAR

Dish of dried figs
(soaked overnight)
Scrambled eggs.
Banana bread; health jam.
Beverage.

SPECIAL

Dish of sliced peaches, apples and
pears; nut-cream dressing.
Soya muffin.
Beverage.

LUNCH

REGULAR

Green salad; french dressing.
Baked potato; vegetable salt,
raw butter or soy margarine.
Steamed string beans.
Pumpkin pudding.
Beverage.

SPECIAL

Tomato stuffed with cottage cheese
and chives on romaine lettuce.
Wheat germ muffins.
Beverage.

DINNER

REGULAR

Vegetable juice.
Lentil curry.
Cole slaw salad.
Date-nut bread with cream cheese.
Beverage.

SPECIAL

Vegetable soup.
Baked potato with yogurt and chives.
Green salad; oil and
lemon dressing.
Fruit honey ice cream.
Beverage.

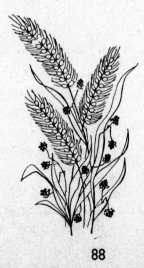

BREAKFAST

1. Fresh fruit juice. Any whole grain cereal with raw milk or goat's milk; raisins, dates or other dried or fresh fruit in season. Honey, molasses or raw sugar may be used for sweetening. Strawberry or prune yogurt may also be used as a topping.

2. Brown rice cooked, raw milk. Sweetening, fruit and yogurt as above.

3. Fresh fruit compote with cottage cheese, yogurt, wheat germ. Beverage (carob milk drink, etc.)

4. Whole wheat pancakes; raw butter; molasses or honey. Beverage.

5. Citrus fruit (2 or 3 oranges or grapefruits) with ½ cup raw nuts or 2 tablespoons nut butter. Beverage.

6. Whole grain dry cereal. Sweetening, fruit and yogurt as in (1).

Children eat REGULAR dinners.

LUNCH-BOX SANDWICHES

1. Nut butter (almond or cashew, raw, unsalted) with health jam or jelly; lemon and honey mixed in; lettuce; whole grain bread. Fruit.

2. Alfalfa sprouts with good quality cream cheese on whole grain bread. Fruit.

3. Blend the following ingredients in blender: 1 avocado, ½ tsp. lemon, ½ tomato, 1 tsp. parsley, 1 green pepper, vegetable salt. Spread on whole grain bread. Fruit.

4. Egg salad made as follows: 2 hard boiled eggs, 1 stalk of celery, 2 tbsp. health food mayonnaise, vegetable salt. Whole grain bread. Fruit.

5. Date-nut cream cheese: ¼ cup dates, ¼ cup nuts, ¼ pack cream cheese (home made if possible). Blend ingredients in blender. Spread on whole grain or banana bread. Fruit.

Use fresh fruit (apples, bananas, pears, etc.) and dried fruits (raisins, dates, figs) for snacks and refreshments between meals.

GREEN SPLIT PEA SOUP

1 cup split peas
1 quart cold water
1 large onion, chopped fine
1 cup celery, diced
2 small carrots, diced
¼ cup parsley, chopped
1 tsp. soya oil
1 tsp. soya sauce (Heatlh Food)
1 tsp. oregano
1 tsp. basil
Vegetable salt to taste.

Soak peas overnight. Simmer peas and vegetables in same water for two hours. Add remaining ingredients. Continue to simmer for one hour or until consistency is smooth. Can be put in blender and pureed. Serves four to six.

VEAL JOINT BROTH

4 lbs. veal joint
1½ cups apple peelings
1½ cups potato peelings
1 celery stalk, chopped
½ cup okra, washed and chopped
1 parsnip, scraped
1 onion, sliced
2 beets, grated
½ cup parsley, chopped
1 bay leaf, if desired
Vegetable salt to taste

Wash veal bone in cold water. Place in large pot. Fill pot half full of water. Bring to boil. Add remaining ingredients. Simmer for four hours. Strain broth.

VEGETABLE SOUP

2 quarts cold water
3 medium carrots, diced
1 medium onion, chopped fine
2 stalks celery, diced
2 medium tomatoes, quartered
¼ pound spinach, chopped
2 medium squash, sliced (summer or zucchini)
1 small cabbage, shredded
2 bouillon cubes
½ tsp. thyme
Vegetable salt to taste

Put all vegetables, except spinach, in water. Add spices and vegetable salt. Simmer until vegetables are partially cooked; about ten minutes. Bouillon cubes and spinach may now be added. Simmer for a few more minutes. Serves four to six.

LENTIL LOAF

1 cup cooked lentils
1 cup bread crumbs
1 cup raw milk
1 egg yolk, beaten
½ cup carrots, scraped and diced
½ cup celery, chopped
¼ cup parsley, chopped
½ tsp. oregano
½ tsp. basil
Vegetable salt to taste
Safflower oil

Mix all ingredients thoroughly. Bake in oiled pan in moderate oven (350 F.) about twenty-five to thirty minutes.

WHOLE WHEAT SPAGHETTI WITH VEGETARIAN SAUCE

6 large tomatoes
2 stalks celery, finely cut
2 small carrots, scraped and diced
½ eggplant, peeled and diced
1 small green pepper, chopped fine
1 medium onion, minced
1 clove garlic, minced
½ tsp. oregano
½ tsp. basil
1 bay leaf, if desired
Vegetable salt to taste
1 lb. whole wheat, soya or spinach spaghetti
3 tbsp. safflower oil
Ricotta or unprocessed cheese

Scald and peel tomatoes. If greater quantity of sauce is desired, use more tomatoes. Saute remaining vegetables in safflower oil. Quarter and add tomatoes. Add seasonings. Simmer about thirty minutes or until desired consistency is reached. Cook spaghetti as directed on package. Drain and blanche. Serve with sauce and sprinkle with cheese. Serves four.

COTTAGE CHEESE DESSERT

1 pound dry cottage cheese
½ cup dried fruit, chopped fine
½ cup unsalted nuts, ground
½ cup raisins, chopped fine
½ cup yogurt
¼ cup raw butter
2 tbsp. honey

Blend ingredients well. Chill. Serve with any fresh fruit.

RICE PUDDING

1 cup brown short grain rice
2 cups raw milk
1 egg, beaten
½ cup brown sugar or honey
¼ cup raisins
½ tsp. cinnamon

Cook rice in two cups of water for forty minutes. Rinse. Mix all ingredients well and place in baking dish. Bake in moderate oven (350 F.) about thirty minutes.

SOYA RICE FLOUR RAISIN BREAD

¼ cup raw milk
2 eggs, beaten
½ cup honey or raw sugar
¼ cup safflower oil
½ cup soya flour
1½ cups brown rice flour
½ tsp. baking soda
1 tsp. baking powder
½ cup raisins
¼ cup nuts (unroasted, unsalted) chopped

Mix milk, eggs, honey and oil. Sift dry ingredients and add slowly. Stir in raisins and nuts. Pour into oiled bread pan. Let stand for one hour. Bake in moderate oven (350 F.) about forty-five minutes. Makes one loaf.

WHEAT GERM MUFFINS

2 eggs, separated
4 tsp. soy oil
1 tsp. honey or raw sugar
1 tsp. salt
1¾ cups raw milk
2 cups whole wheat flour, sifted
1 cup wheat germ
1 tsp. baking powder
¼ cup raisins

Beat egg yolks until thick and creamy. Stir in oil, honey and salt. Slowly add milk. Blend in flour, wheat germ and baking powder. Add raisins. Beat egg whites until stiff. Fold into mixture. Pour into well oiled muffin tins. Bake in moderate oven (350 F.) about thirty minutes. Makes one dozen.

DRINKS

some using brewers yeast or wheat germ powder

Brewers yeast is the most commonly accepted natural source for the B Vitamin group. Two tablespoonfuls (1 ounce) would contain the following approximate amount of the B Vitamins:

B_1	4. mg.
B_2	1.2 mg.
Niacin	11. mg.

Plus other trace factors of Vitamin B-6 and B-12 as naturally found present in brewers yeast.

Wheat germ, the embryo of a kernel of wheat, is a concentrated source of protein, iron, Vitamin E, and the B Vitamins. Two tablespoonfuls (1 ounce) of wheat germ powder would contain the following approximate values:

Calories	30.8		Iron	.7	mg.
Protein	2.1	grms.	Vit. E	7.5	mg.
Fat	.9	grms.	Vit. B_1	.17	mg.
Carbohydrate	4.25	grms.	Vit. B_2	.066	mg.
Calcium	7.1	mg.	Niacin	.4	mg.

Plus other trace factors naturally present in wheat germ powder. (All 8 essential amino acids)

GRAPE-APPLE DRINK (2 cups)

½ cup grape juice
1 cup apple juice
2 tsp. brewers yeast
1 tbsp. yogurt
¼ cup raisins

Blend

PINEAPPLE DRINK (2 cups)

1½ cups pineapple juice
1 ripe banana
1 tbsp. yogurt
2 tsp. wheat germ powder
1 tsp sunflower meal

Blend

FRUIT JUICE DRINK (1 CUP)

¼ cup papaya juice
¼ cup orange juice
¼ cup pineapple juice
cup coconut juice

Mix or blend

DATE NUT SHAKE (2 CUPS)

1 cup raw or non-fat milk
½ cup dates (pitted)
1 tbsp. nut butter
1 tbsp. carob powder

Blend in blender

CARROT MILK DRINK (1 cup)

½ cup carrot juice
½ cup certified raw milk
¼ cup almonds chopped
2 tsp. wheat germ powder

Blend

PINEAPPLE-COCONUT DRINK (1 cup)

½ cup coconut juice
½ cup pineapple juice
1 tsp. powdered wheat germ
1 tbsp. yogurt

Blend or mix well

TOMATO DRINK (1 cup)

1 cup tomato juice
1 tsp. parsley chopped
1 tsp. lemon juice
2 tsp. brewers yeast

Blend

APPLE JUICE DRINK (1 cup)

1 cup apple juice
1 tbsp. yogurt
1 to 2 tsp. brewers yeast
1 drop pure vanilla extract

Blend or mix well

TOMATO-SAUERKRAUT DRINK (1 cup)

½ cup tomato juice
½ cup sauerkraut juice
1 tsp. parsley chopped
2 tsp. brewers yeast

Blend

CARROT-COCONUT DRINK (1 cup)

½ cup carrot juice
¼ cup celery juice
¼ cup coconut juice
1 tsp. parsley chopped
1 tsp. brewers yeast

Blend

WEIGHT GAINING DRINK (2 cups)

1 cup orange juice
1 tsp. safflower oil
1 tbsp. carrot ice cream
1 egg
1 tbsp. brewers yeast
1 tsp. cashew nut butter

Liquify in blender

VEGETABLE DRINK (2 cups)

½ cup tomato juice
¼ cup celery juice
¼ cup carrot juice
¼ bunch water cress chopped
1 tsp. parsley chopped
1 tsp. lemon juice
2 tsp. brewers yeast

Blend

CAROB DRINK (1 cup)

1 cup certified raw milk
1 tbsp. carob powder
1 egg yolk
1 tsp. wheat germ powder
1 drop pure vanilla extract

Blend

PINEAPPLE-CARROT DRINK (1 cup)

½ cup pineapple juice
½ cup carrot juice
1 tsp. lemon juice
1 tsp. shredded coconut
2 tsp. brewers yeast

Blend

FRUIT MILK DRINK (1 cup)

½ cup raw or non-fat milk
½ cup any fruit juice
½ tsp. honey (or more if desired)

Mix or blend

ENERGY DRINK (1½ CUPS)

½ cup prune juice
½ cup apple juice
1 tsp. nut butter
1 tsp. yogurt
1 tsp. soy, sesame or
   safflower oil

Blend in blender

CAROB MILK DRINK (3 CUPS)

2 cups raw certified milk
   (or non-fat milk)
2 tbsp. carob powder
1 tbsp. honey or molasses
1 banana
1 tbsp. nut butter

Blend

POTASSIUM (VEGETABLE) DRINK
(2 CUPS)

¼ cup parsley juice
¼ cup carrot juice
¼ cup celery juice
¼ cup watercress
¼ cup spinach

Mix or blend

DATE MILK (1 cup)

1 cup certified raw milk
3 dates chopped
1 tbsp. shredded coconut
1 tsp. wheat germ powder
1 tsp. safflower oil

Blend

GRAPE JUICE DRINK (1½ CUPS)

1 cup grape juice (unsweetened)
1 tbsp. brewers yeast
½ tbsp. sunflower meal
1 tbsp. yogurt
1 tsp. carob powder

Blend in blender

VEGETABLE JUICE DRINK (1 CUP)

⅓ cup carrot juice
⅓ cup celery juice
⅓ cup tomato juice
1 tbsp. brewers yeast

Mix well or blend in blender

FRUIT JUICE-EGG DRINK (1½ CUP)

½ cup orange juice
½ cup papaya juice
1 egg
1 tsp. honey

Mix or blend

VEGETABLE-FRUIT JUICE DRINK (2 cups).

½ cup carrot juice
½ cup papaya or coconut juice
1 banana
1 tbsp. wheat germ
2 dates (pitted)

Mix well or blend in blender

VEGETABLE JUICE DRINK (1 CUP)

⅓ cup beet juice
⅓ cup cucumber juice
⅓ carrot juice
1 tbsp. brewers yeast

Mix well or blend in blender

BEVERAGES

All Fresh Fruit and Vegetable Juices
Vegetable Broths
Herb Teas
Cereal Beverages (coffee substitutes)

OILS

Safflower Oil
Sesame Seed Oil
Pure Olive Oil
(use for cooking and dressings)

MINERALS (this last includes most fruits and vegetables)

Apples, Apricots, Artichokes, Beets, Blueberries, Broccoli, Brussels Sprouts, Cabbage, Cauliflower, Carrots, Celery, Cherries, Cranberries, Cucumbers, Dandelion, Eggplant, Endive, Garlic, Grapes, Grapefruit, Green Peas, Green Peppers, Kale, Leeks, Lemons, Limes, Lettuce, Melons, Mustard Greens, Oranges, Parsley, Parsnips, Peaches, Pears, Pineapples, Plums, Pomegranates, Prunes, Radishes, Raspberries, Rhubarb, Spinach, Strawberries, String Beans, Squash, Tangerines, Tomatoes, Turnips, Watercress.

DAIRY FOODS

Goat Milk
Certified Raw Milk
Non-fat Milk
Yogurt (and all sour milk products)
Cottage Cheese (uncreamed)
Farmer Cheese
Ricotta Cheese (and Italian cheese)
Butter (made from whole milk)
(buttermilk and sour cream not suggested)

PROTEINS

Avocados
Legumes (beans, peas, lentils, soy beans and soy bean products)
Nuts (unroasted and unsalted; almonds, cashews, pecans, walnuts, brazil nuts; not peanuts)
Coconuts (and coconut milk)
Nut Butters (almond, cashew; not peanut)
Meat (organ meat preferred, particularly beef liver, kidneys, brains)
Poultry (very moderately)
Fish (that live on sea vegetables)
See also "Dairy Foods"

STARCHES

Bananas
Brown Rice
Potatoes (baked, boiled)
Whole Grain Breads, Crackers
Pumpkin
Barley
Rye

GRAINS

All Whole Grain products
(no refined flour products)

CONDIMENTS

All edible Herbs
Vegetable salt

SUGARS

All Fresh Fruits
Molasses
Honey (uncooked, unblended)
Raw Sugar
Beet Sugar
Cane Sugar (the cane stalks)
Carob (St. John's Bread)
Dried Fruits: Dates, Figs, Prunes, Raisin
Apricots, Peaches, etc.